The Lyme Disease 30-Day Meal Plan

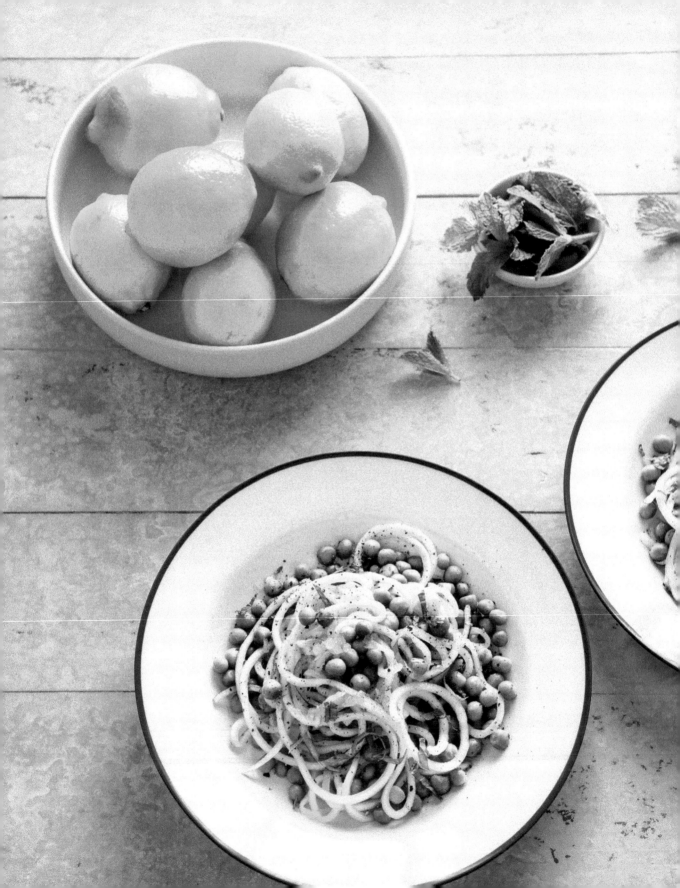

The LYME DISEASE

30-Day Meal Plan

HEALTHY RECIPES AND LIFESTYLE TIPS TO EASE SYMPTOMS

Lindsay Christensen, M.S.

ROCKRIDGE
PRESS

Interior and Cover Designer: Will Mack
Art Manager: Karen Beard
Editor: Marisa A. Hines
Production Manager: Riley Hoffman
Production Editor: Melissa Edeburn

Cover and interior photography ©Nadine Greeff, except pg. 2 ©Aleksandr Kutakh/Shutterstock. Author photo courtesy of Bergreen Photography.

ISBN: Print 978-1-64152-556-5 | eBook 978-1-64152-557-2

*To my parents, Mark and Laura Christensen;
without your unconditional love and support,
I would not be where I am today.*

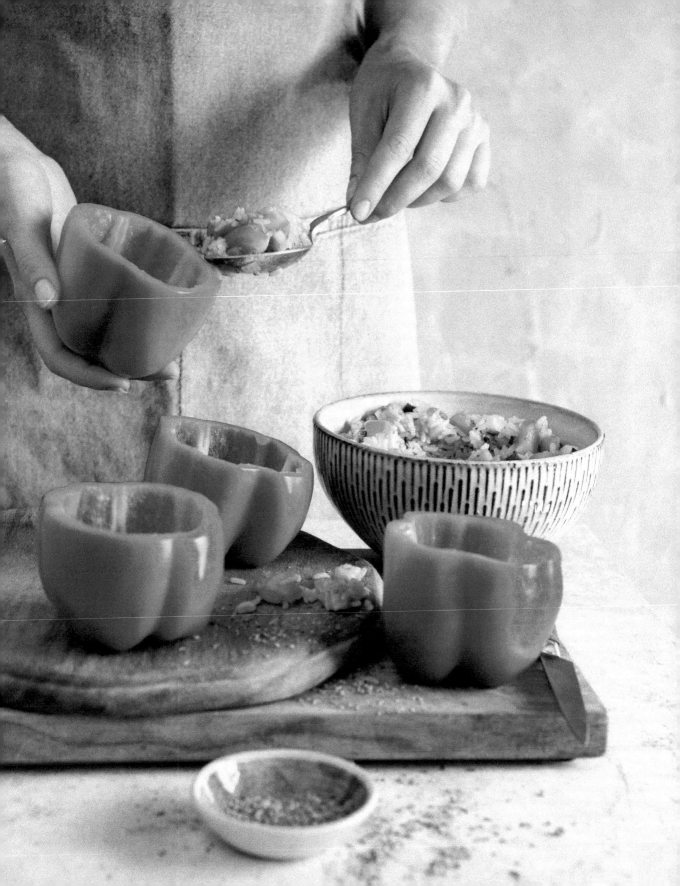

Contents

Introduction

In 2010, as a healthy college undergrad with the world before me, I could never have imagined the path my life would take over the next 10 years. Upon entering freshman year, a time that, for most students, includes socializing and discovering yourself, I became severely ill with a mysterious illness that left me struggling with insomnia, strange rashes, tremors, brain fog, and chronic fatigue. As an inquisitive and extremely driven pre-med student, I was dissatisfied with the explanations given to me by my doctors, who largely believed my symptoms were the result of "stress." Over the course of several years in my late teens and early twenties, I visited more than 30 different healthcare professionals, never ceasing my quest to understand what had gone wrong with my body and how I could fix it.

When I was finally given a diagnosis of chronic Lyme disease at the age of 22, I was, at first, greatly relieved. Finally, I had an answer as to why I was so sick! Little did I know that this diagnosis was nowhere near the end of my journey; in fact, it simply marked the beginning of a new one—that of learning how to recover from Lyme disease. Over the next four years I set out to learn and consume everything I could get my hands on about Lyme disease and how to improve my symptoms. This journey led me to realize that health is not something to be taken for granted; rather, it is something that we must work for consistently each and every day of our lives. Diet and lifestyle changes are two areas in which you can work to improve your health daily. Making healthy diet and lifestyle changes is particularly important if you have been diagnosed with Lyme disease.

The axiom "You are what you eat" is especially true for Lyme disease patients. Research indicates that the foods we choose to eat have a profound impact on our bodies, influencing everything from immunity to brain function. A healthy diet can help reduce Lyme disease symptoms by alleviating chronic inflammation, boosting energy production, and fortifying the immune system. In my personal journey with Lyme disease and my clinical nutrition practice, I have witnessed the great benefits proper nutrition can have in the context of Lyme disease. Simple dietary changes helped me regain my energy, banish brain fog, and strengthen my immune system, greatly reducing the impact of Lyme on my life. On the basis of my personal and clinical experiences, I firmly believe that diet and lifestyle changes should be central in any treatment plan for Lyme disease.

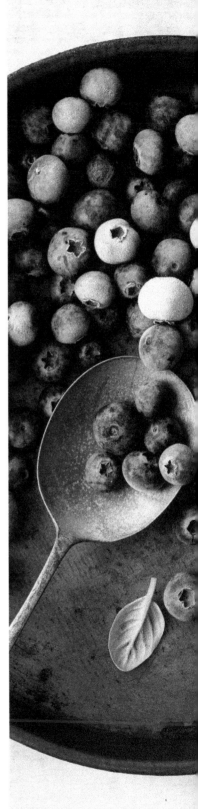

Regarding nutrition, many conflicting opinions are presented on the Internet and in the media. For the Lyme disease patient suffering from brain fog and extreme fatigue, the idea of having to sort through all this information can be overwhelming, to say the least. My goal is to offer a concise nutritional plan, backed by scientific research and clinical experience, that removes the burden of identifying useful information for yourself amid the confusing mass of articles and advice available online and on TV.

In this book, you will find a handy food list detailing which foods to consume and which to avoid, plus grocery shopping tips and a trove of recipes for healthy, satisfying meals that are both delicious and easy to prepare. These recipes will nourish your body without drawing excessively on your energy reserves and time. I have also selected recipes with ingredients that are natural and wholesome, yet affordable.

This book contains the cumulative knowledge I have gathered over the years about nutrition and lifestyle changes that promote recovery from Lyme disease. Although these changes are not a cure for Lyme disease, they may help you navigate your way to a healthier life.

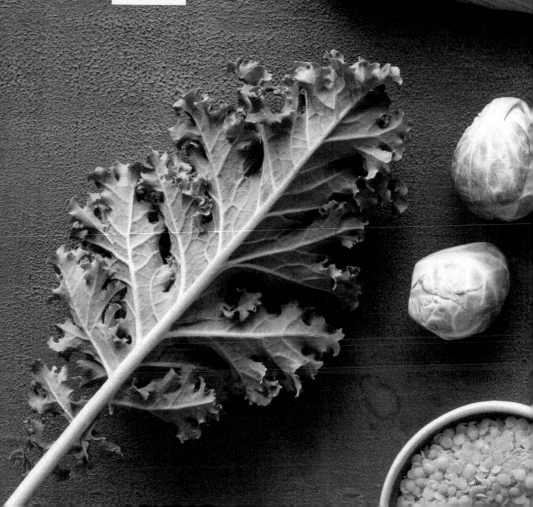

PART 1

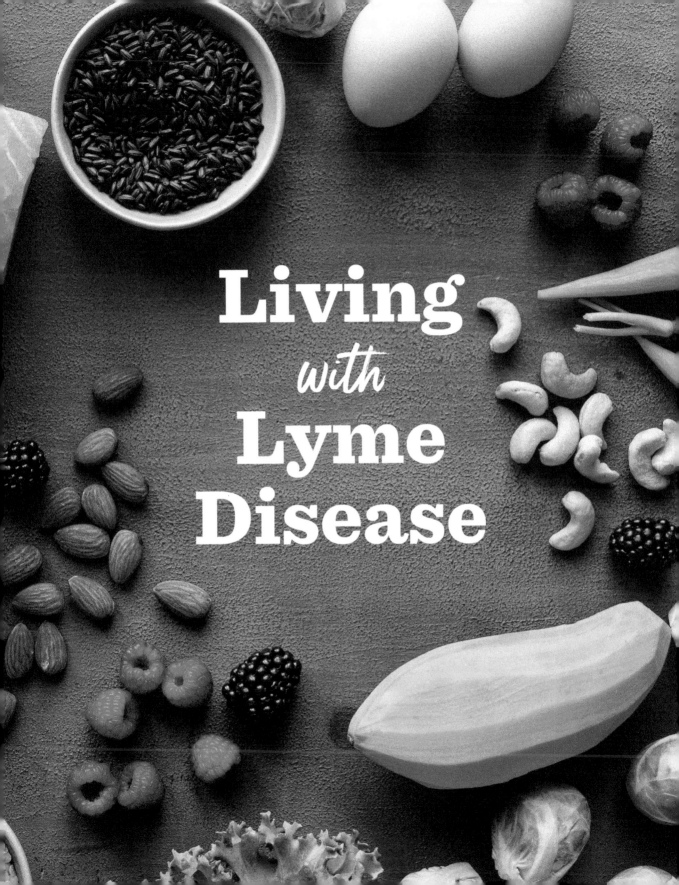

Living

with

Lyme
Disease

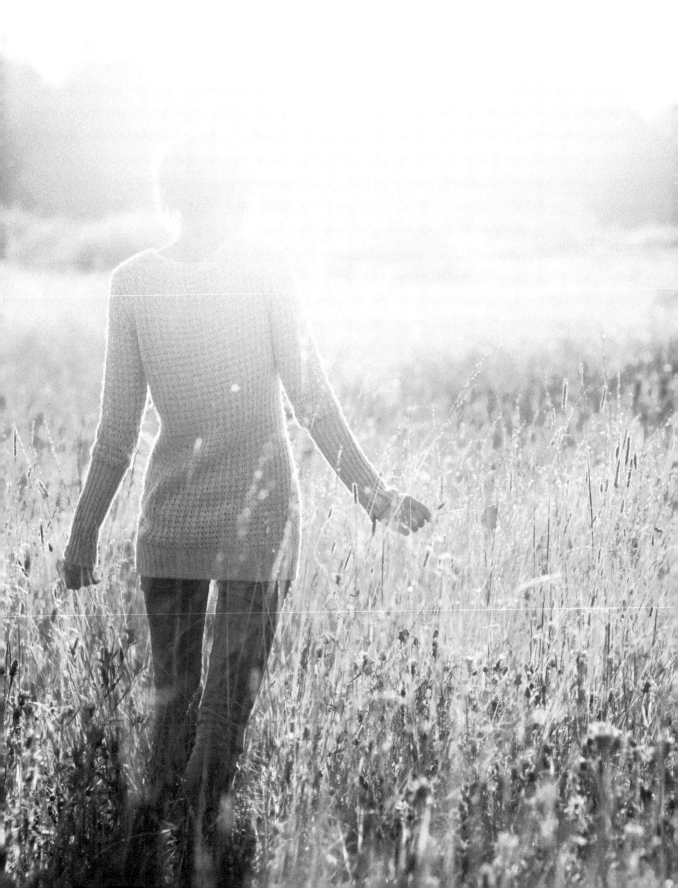

Chapter 1

Understanding Lyme Disease

Lyme disease is one of the fastest-growing infectious diseases in the United States. Recent surveys of commercial laboratories indicate that a shocking 300,000 Americans are diagnosed with the disease each year; although large, this number vastly underrepresents the true prevalence of Lyme disease due to underreporting, inaccurate testing, and the fact that many patients with suspected Lyme disease undergo treatment without testing. Experts in the medical and scientific communities have gone so far as to deem Lyme disease an epidemic and public health crisis. Despite the growing prevalence of Lyme disease, many people (physicians and laypeople alike) believe that it only affects animals or that it is rare in humans. Unfortunately, this notion couldn't be further from the truth. So what exactly is Lyme disease? Who is susceptible, and how can you determine whether Lyme is affecting you? Let's begin with the basics.

What Is Lyme Disease?

Lyme disease is an inflammatory tick-borne disease that was first discovered in 1975 in the town of Old Lyme, Connecticut. In this town, a group of children and adults were suffering from puzzling and debilitating health issues, including swollen knees, skin rashes, headaches, chronic fatigue, and paralysis. The U.S. government called in clinicians and scientists to study the group's symptoms. They soon ascertained that all the affected children had been bitten by ticks prior to the onset of their symptoms. The researchers named the condition Lyme disease. The cause of the disease, a bacterium called *Borrelia burgdorferi*, was identified several years later, in 1981, by scientist Willy Burgdorfer.

Since the 1980s, the incidence of Lyme disease has increased dramatically across the United States and around the world. Although Lyme disease was once considered to be limited to the northeastern United States, it has since been identified in all 50 states and in 80 other countries. The exploding rates of Lyme disease have forced scientists and healthcare providers to evolve their understanding of the disease process. It is now understood that ticks transmit dozens of pathogens besides *Borrelia burgdorferi*, including other types of bacteria, parasites, and viruses. These pathogens transmitted simultaneously with *Borrelia* are referred to as "coinfections." This phenomenon makes Lyme disease far more complex than previously believed.

Telltale bullseye and other common symptoms

Historically, health authorities have associated Lyme disease with a set of common symptoms. These symptoms include a telltale bullseye rash, fever, flu-like symptoms, fatigue and malaise, and joint stiffness and swelling.

The telltale bullseye rash is perhaps the manifestation of Lyme disease most popularized by the media. This skin irritation typically appears on the limbs or trunk of the body of an infected individual and does indeed resemble a bullseye. However, statistics indicate that only 19 percent of Lyme-associated rashes are a true bullseye rash. Therefore, it is entirely possible to be infected with *Borrelia burgdorferi* despite never experiencing a bullseye rash. Unfortunately, atypical (non-bullseye) rashes caused by Lyme are frequently mistaken for a skin infection or spider bite, which prevents an accurate diagnosis.

It is crucial to note that these common symptoms of Lyme disease are most often experienced in the acute stages of the infection. Patients who receive a late diagnosis or who have chronic (persistent) Lyme (see page 14) experience different and often more severe symptoms.

Who is susceptible?

Contrary to previously held beliefs, Lyme disease does not just afflict people living in the northeastern United States. Anyone who has had contact with a tick can contract Lyme disease. Children, the elderly, and those who work outdoors tend to be most susceptible to the disease. However, susceptibility also varies widely from one person to another due to differences in age, genetics, and immune status.

Why Lyme disease is difficult to diagnose

Lyme disease is notoriously difficult to diagnose for four reasons:

- Many people with symptoms of Lyme disease do not recall experiencing a tick bite.

- Lyme disease mimics other health conditions.

- Ticks that spread Lyme disease also spread other diseases that can complicate the clinical picture.

- The standard lab tests endorsed by the Centers for Disease Control and Prevention (CDC) for the diagnosis of Lyme disease are only intended to diagnose acute, not chronic, Lyme disease. Furthermore, they frequently give false negatives, leading people to believe they don't have Lyme when, in fact, they do have the disease.

Many physicians are still under the assumption that Lyme disease is contracted either immediately after a tick bite or not at all. **However, a growing body of research indicates that many people infected with *Borrelia burgdorferi* do not recall experiencing a tick bite.** A recent study published in *Ticks and Tick-borne Diseases* found that only a minority of children with confirmed Lyme disease had a recognized tick bite, leading the authors to conclude that "lack of a tick bite history does not reliably exclude Lyme disease."

To complicate matters further, people who do experience a tick bite may initially be asymptomatic and then experience a flare of symptoms several months later. Unfortunately, the possibility of Lyme disease is often dismissed in these cases, and patients are instead misdiagnosed with conditions that have symptoms resembling those of late-stage Lyme, such as rheumatoid arthritis, Sjogren's syndrome, or, in extreme cases, Alzheimer's disease.

Another significant barrier to the timely diagnosis of Lyme disease is created by the testing methods currently endorsed by the CDC and the Infectious Diseases Society of America (IDSA): the ELISA and Western Blot tests. The ELISA (enzyme-linked immunosorbent assay) is the screening test used when Lyme disease is first suspected. It measures the levels of antibodies against *Borrelia burgdorferi*. (Antibodies are large proteins used by the immune system to neutralize pathogens such as bacteria and viruses.) According to the CDC, if an ELISA for *Borrelia burgdorferi* is negative, no further testing for Lyme disease is needed; if the ELISA is positive, a second test is recommended to confirm the presence of disease. However, concerning statistics indicate that the ELISA produces false negatives 50 percent of the time, leading many people to believe they don't have the disease when, in fact, they do.

The Western Blot is typically run as a second-stage test to confirm a positive ELISA test for Lyme disease. It reports reactivity against 10 different proteins found on *Borrelia burgdorferi*; according to the CDC, five of these bands must be positive in order to produce a Western Blot positive for Lyme disease. This test is generally more reliable than ELISA. Unfortunately, however, many doctors do not use this test unless an ELISA is positive, thereby missing many Lyme diagnoses.

The combined sensitivity of the CDC's two-tiered testing strategy in the early stages of Lyme is pretty dismal, at approximately 30 to 40 percent. This means the ELISA and Western Blot only correctly identify those with acute Lyme disease 30 to 40 percent of the time! For all stages of Lyme disease, acute and chronic, the combined sensitivity only increases slightly, to 57.6 percent.

When to Talk with Your Doctor

If you have been exposed to a tick or are experiencing any of the symptoms of Lyme disease mentioned on page 4, it is time to talk with your doctor. If you are bitten by a tick, record the initial bite date and symptoms. Next, remove the tick and preserve it. This step is crucial because the tick can then be sent to a special laboratory that can determine what pathogens, if any, it is carrying; this information will help your doctor make treatment decisions.

Take the following steps to safely remove and preserve a tick at home:

1. Remove the tick promptly and carefully. Use fine-tipped tweezers or a special tick-removal tool, such as the TickEase Tweezers, and grasp the tick close to the skin. Pull the tick out using a slow and steady motion. Avoid squeezing or twisting the tick, as this may cause part of it to break off in your skin. Do not use petroleum jelly, a hot match, or any other items to remove the tick.

2. Seal the tick in a container, such as a Ziploc bag or Tupperware container. Place the container in the freezer.

3. Wash your hands and the bite site with soap and water.

Preparing for your visit

Once you have an appointment scheduled with your doctor, there are a few things you should do to prepare.

❏ **Bring copies of all your medical test results.** Bring a copy of the results from every medical test you've undergone since the onset of your symptoms. These lab reports will help your doctor put together the pieces of your health puzzle and determine whether further testing is needed.

❏ **Create a list of your symptoms.** Each symptom you are experiencing is a clue your doctor can use to determine whether your sickness is indeed caused by Lyme, or by one of the other conditions that frequently accompany Lyme disease, such as coinfections or mold illness. The brain fog common in Lyme patients may make it difficult for you to remember all of your symptoms on the spot; having a list handy will help you make the most of your appointment with your doctor.

❏ **Bring a list of current medications and supplements and their dosages.** A number of nutritional supplements and herbs can potentially interact with pharmaceutical drugs, decreasing their effectiveness or increasing their toxicity. Providing your doctor with a list of your current medications and supplements can help prevent adverse drug-supplement interactions.

❏ **Bring an outline of your overall health.** Providing your doctor with a "health timeline" can help him or her increase the accuracy of your diagnosis.

❏ **Write down your questions.** Writing down these questions ahead of time will save you the frustration of trying to remember all of your questions during your appointment. Here are the top five questions you may want to ask your doctor:

- What testing do you recommend?
- What kind of symptoms can I expect during antibiotic treatment?
- What should I expect after taking the antibiotics?
- Are there things I can do to support my body during antibiotic treatment?
- What will we do next if antibiotic treatment doesn't work?

During your visit

During the visit with your doctor, he or she will first conduct a physical exam. Your doctor should follow this with an order for an ELISA test and Western Blot. In some cases, if Lyme disease is strongly suspected, a doctor may write a prescription for a course of antibiotics right off the bat, before getting the results of the ELISA and Western Blot.

Going into a doctor's appointment to discuss the possibility of Lyme disease can be overwhelming. To make the most of your visit, take the following steps:

Bring a friend or family member with you to your appointment. This person may remember aspects of your health journey that have slipped your mind but are crucial for helping your doctor understand your illness and provide the correct diagnosis.

Don't be afraid to ask questions. The possibility of having Lyme disease is a frightening proposition for many people, and it's likely that you have many questions. Your doctor's role is to provide you with the highest quality care possible, which includes answering your questions. As I mentioned previously, bring a list of your questions to your appointment so you don't forget anything.

Bring photos of any previous suspicious rashes and copies of all your lab work. Providing your doctor with these items will help him or her better piece together your health puzzle and create a customized treatment protocol.

Find out whether you may contact your doctor after the appointment if you have more questions. Oftentimes, we think of additional questions immediately after a doctor's appointment; this is why it is helpful to have a doctor who is reachable between appointments. A growing number of doctors offer between-appointment support via e-mail or in the form of HIPAA-compliant patient portals.

The benefits of working with a Lyme-literate doctor

Unfortunately, doctors are often misinformed about Lyme disease. Many believe that the disease can only be contracted in the northeastern United States, and that you must have the telltale bullseye rash or other common symptoms to warrant a diagnosis of Lyme disease. **If your doctor is dismissive of your concerns about Lyme disease, seek out a Lyme-literate doctor instead.** Lyme-literate doctors (LLMDs) have received special training in Lyme disease diagnosis and treatment. They are, therefore, far more informed about Lyme disease than the average physician. The International Lyme and Associated Diseases Society (ILADS) and Global Lyme Alliance (GLA) both offer physician directories on their websites where you can search for a Lyme-literate doctor in your area.

Early Diagnosis

What is an early diagnosis?

A diagnosis of Lyme is considered "early" when it is made a few weeks after a tick bite; several weeks' time is needed for the body to mount an immune response to *Borrelia burgdorferi*, producing antibodies that can be detected by the ELISA and Western Blot. Catching Lyme disease early and promptly treating it can significantly reduce your chances of experiencing complications down the road. However, as previously mentioned, the ELISA and Western Blot are not perfect; it is possible to test for and miss Lyme disease even in the early stages. If your ELISA or Western Blot comes back negative but you strongly suspect Lyme disease, be persistent. Find a doctor willing to test you again and realize that it can take four to six weeks for Lyme tests to come back positive, even in the acute stages of infection.

Early diagnosis symptoms

The most common symptoms of early-stage Lyme disease are rashes, fever, chills, headache, swollen lymph nodes, stiff neck, fatigue, and muscle and joint pain. Atypical rashes, or rashes other than the telltale bullseye rash, are common and may appear as uniform red, disseminated, blistering, and/or blue-red lesions on the skin. Though typically associated with the later stages of Lyme disease, neurological symptoms such as numbness, paralysis of the facial muscles, and visual disturbances can also signify early-stage Lyme disease.

COMMON EARLY SYMPTOMS

Have you recently been bitten by a tick? The following symptoms are a sign that you may be infected with Lyme disease.

Rashes: Although the classic bullseye rash is the most well-known skin manifestation of Lyme disease, *Borrelia burgdorferi* can also trigger other rashes, including uniform red patches, blistering lesions, disseminated lesions, and blue-red lesions on the skin.

Fever: Fever is a common early-stage symptom of Lyme disease. It is frequently accompanied by other flu-like symptoms, such as chills.

Night sweats: Night sweats are a common side effect of many bacterial infections, including Lyme disease.

Headache: Have you suddenly developed cluster headaches or migraines? When accompanied by some of the other symptoms discussed here, headaches can indicate a Lyme infection. These headaches are caused by the inflammatory response *Borrelia burgdorferi* induces in the neurological system.

Fatigue: Do you normally lead a busy, active life, but suddenly can't seem to rouse yourself from the couch? Sudden, severe fatigue and malaise are indicators that you may have Lyme disease.

Stiff neck: Infection with *Borrelia burgdorferi* causes inflammation of the protective tissues covering the brain and spinal cord called the meninges. When these tissues are inflamed, neck pain may result.

Swollen lymph nodes: The lymphatic system is your body's first-line defense against pathogens, including *Borrelia burgdorferi*. The proliferation of immune system molecules in response to *Borrelia* can cause your lymph nodes, located behind your ears, under your jawline, and in your armpits and groin, to swell and feel tender. When you see your doctor, he or she should palpate your lymph nodes to determine whether they are swollen.

Muscle and joint pain: Are you normally a very physically active person, but have suddenly begun to experience knee pain or joint stiffness? When accompanied by the other symptoms mentioned here, a sudden onset of muscle and joint pain and stiffness is suggestive of Lyme disease.

Treatment options

The standard of care endorsed by the CDC and IDSA for Lyme disease is a course of antibiotics. Treatment may come in the form of a 14- to 21-day course of oral antibiotics or a 14- to 28-day course of intravenous antibiotics. Alternative medications have not been scientifically proven to be effective for treating early Lyme disease.

If you are fortunate enough to get an early diagnosis, a course of antibiotics may be sufficient to eradicate the infection. **It should be noted, however, that a growing body of research indicates that the standard antibiotic approach does not work for *all people* diagnosed with early Lyme disease.** Studies show that *Borrelia burgdorferi* infection can persist even after the standard 28-day course of antibiotics. If you receive an early diagnosis of Lyme disease, undergo the standard course of treatment, and feel worse or experience a return of your symptoms upon stopping antibiotic treatment, you may need continuing care to treat the infection.

Late Diagnosis

What is a late diagnosis?

A late diagnosis of Lyme disease occurs when the initial symptoms of infection were not present or caught in time, leading to the development of secondary conditions. **In late Lyme disease, *Borrelia burgdorferi* has disseminated from the original site of infection to other parts of the body.** It then begins to induce an inflammatory response in these body parts, leading to the symptoms of late Lyme disease.

Late diagnosis symptoms

When *Borrelia burgdorferi* becomes disseminated in late Lyme disease, it induces inflammation and dysfunction in multiple body systems, including the central nervous system, cardiovascular system, and musculoskeletal system. **Unlike the symptoms of early Lyme disease, the symptoms of late Lyme disease are vague, making the condition more difficult to diagnose.** Symptoms of late Lyme disease include the following:

Rashes: Rashes, referred to as *erythema migrans*, may appear on other parts of the body besides the initial site of infection.

Joint and Muscle Pain: This pain is caused by the inflammatory response induced in joints and muscles by disseminated *Borrelia burgdorferi*.

Fatigue: An overall feeling of exhaustion despite adequate rest can be a sign of Lyme infection.

Neurological problems: Neurological issues including inflammation of the membranes surrounding the brain and spinal cord, paralysis of one side of the face, numbness and weakness of the limbs, impaired muscle movement, and memory issues can occur weeks, months, and even years after the initial infection.

Potential health coverage issues

In order for Lyme disease to be medically recognized, the CDC relies on signs of specific organ damage confirmed by a positive Western Blot for antibodies to *Borrelia burgdorferi*. However, this blood test only checks for your immune system's response to the bacteria, not for the presence of the bacteria itself. This method of testing can produce false negatives because it can take weeks for your immune system to respond to *Borrelia*. Unfortunately, false negatives result in a lack of laboratory proof of the disease and may, therefore, prevent you from getting health insurance coverage for treatment.

Treatment options

Unlike in the early stage of Lyme disease, antibiotics are not necessarily beneficial in the later stages of the disease and may come with significant risks. Currently, there is no single course of action determined to be useful for late-stage Lyme disease patients. In this situation, you will need to be your own best advocate. Seek out a doctor familiar with late Lyme disease. He or she may recommend a course of antibiotics complemented by additional, alternative supportive treatments such as botanical medicine. The most important thing is that you do not leave Lyme disease untreated. If late-stage Lyme disease is left untreated, it can progress further and seriously compromise the musculoskeletal, neurological, and cardiovascular systems.

LATER DIAGNOSIS TESTS TO REQUEST

Multiple tests claim to be useful for the diagnosis of late-stage and chronic Lyme disease. According to the CDC, the tests for diagnosing late-stage and chronic Lyme are the same as those for early Lyme disease: the ELISA and, if that comes back positive, the Western Blot. Unfortunately, these tests produce false negatives in many patients with late-stage and chronic Lyme. The ELISA and Western Blot should still be ordered in suspected cases of Lyme disease, though the following tests should also be considered:

IGeneX: This biotechnology company offers advanced, state-of-the-art testing for Lyme disease and Lyme coinfections. Its ImmunoBlot test is a highly sensitive alternative to the traditional Western Blot test.

Polymerase chain reaction (PCR): This DNA test is an important diagnostic tool for patients who have received negative blood tests but still strongly suspect Lyme disease. It requires taking specimens from different body compartments, such as the blood serum and joint fluid.

ArminLabs: This company offers innovative alternatives to the ELISA and Western Blot tests, including EliSpot, which assesses the T-cell immune response to *Borrelia burgdorferi*, thus reflecting current Lyme activity.

Disclaimer: Before initiating a test, contact your insurance provider to understand what can and can't be covered so you can understand your out-of-pocket costs.

Chronic (Persistent) Lyme Disease (CLD)

What is CLD?

Chronic (persistent) Lyme disease (CLD) occurs when a person who's been diagnosed with Lyme disease and treated with antibiotics continues to experience disease symptoms. Although the medical community has debated the existence of CLD for decades, mounting evidence indicates that CLD is a distinct disease entity experienced by approximately 10 to 20 percent of people who have previously been diagnosed with Lyme and treated with antibiotics. Importantly, CLD is often identified in people who don't recall experiencing a tick bite but have multiple, unremitting symptoms of the disease.

Chronic symptoms

The symptoms of chronic Lyme disease are similar to those of late Lyme disease, but they may be more severe. These symptoms include rashes, joint and muscle pain, paresthesia, cognitive dysfunction, fatigue, and sleep disturbances. Gut dysfunction, cardiovascular abnormalities, and severe psychiatric changes, such as depression and suicidality, may also occur. A growing body of research indicates that chronic Lyme disease may also contribute to the development of autoimmune diseases by impairing normal immune system function.

Why does Lyme disease become chronic?

Borrelia burgdorferi is a tricky organism; it has evolved complex mechanisms that allow it to evade its host's immune system. The spiral-shaped *Borrelia burgdorferi* will actually burrow into the organs of its host, inciting organ dysfunction.

Potential health coverage issues

Unfortunately, chronic Lyme disease is still not recognized by most medical professionals. This is despite the fact that a growing body of research indicates that CLD is a legitimate health condition that seriously impacts the function and quality of life of thousands of people. Only a small minority of physicians recognize CLD—many of these physicians are Lyme-literate doctors. Most of these doctors are less likely to prescribe long-term antibiotics; instead, they may use short-term antibiotics alongside botanical medicines and nutrition and detoxification support.

Treatment options

There is no single effective medical treatment for CLD. If you have CLD and choose to work with a Lyme-literate doctor, he or she will most likely use a combination of alternative interventions to create your treatment plan. Even though these treatments can significantly alleviate symptoms of Lyme disease and restore your health, they are rarely covered by insurance and are, therefore, mostly out-of-pocket expenses.

POST-TREATMENT LYME DISEASE SYNDROME

According to the CDC, post-treatment Lyme disease syndrome (PTLDS) is a condition in which nonspecific symptoms such as fatigue and joint pain persist after Lyme disease has been treated with antibiotics. In 2017, Johns Hopkins University researchers published a study showing that PTLDS is "a real disorder that causes severe symptoms in the absence of clinically detectable infection." Scientists speculate that the symptoms of PTLDS may be the result of an aberrant immune response left over from the original infection.

Extended antibiotic therapy, sometimes for longer than six months, has been proposed as treatment for PTLDS. However, research shows that this approach causes significant harm to patients. The conventional medical system does not have a good answer as to how PTLDS should be treated. However, going a more holistic route with the help of a Lyme-literate doctor may go a long way in helping relieve the symptoms of PTLDS.

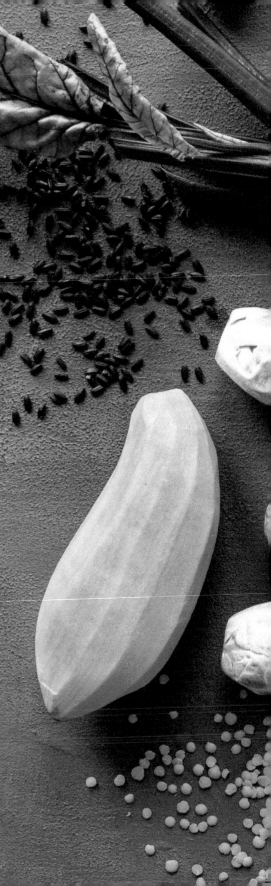

PART 2

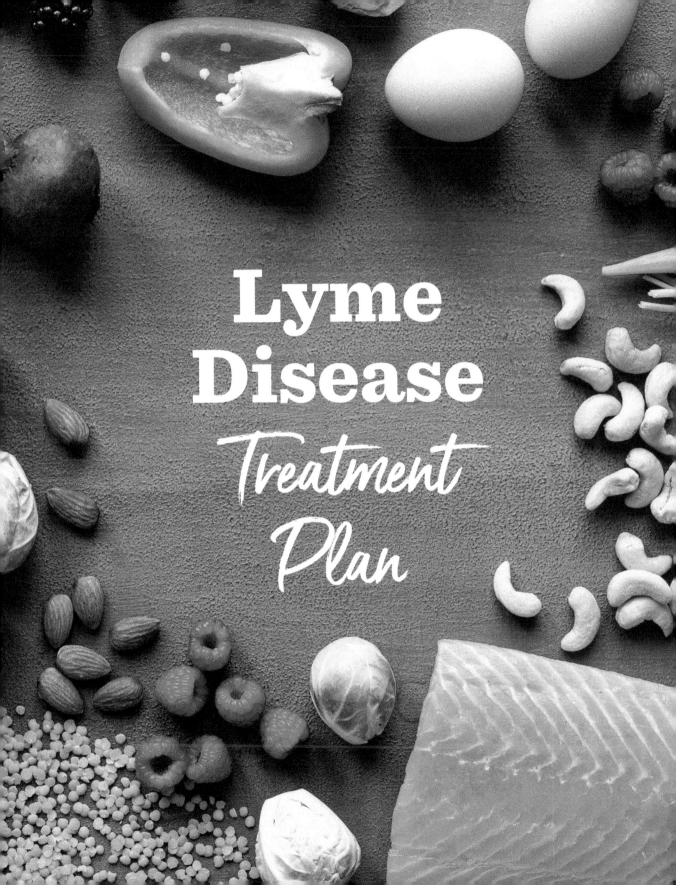

Lyme Disease

Treatment Plan

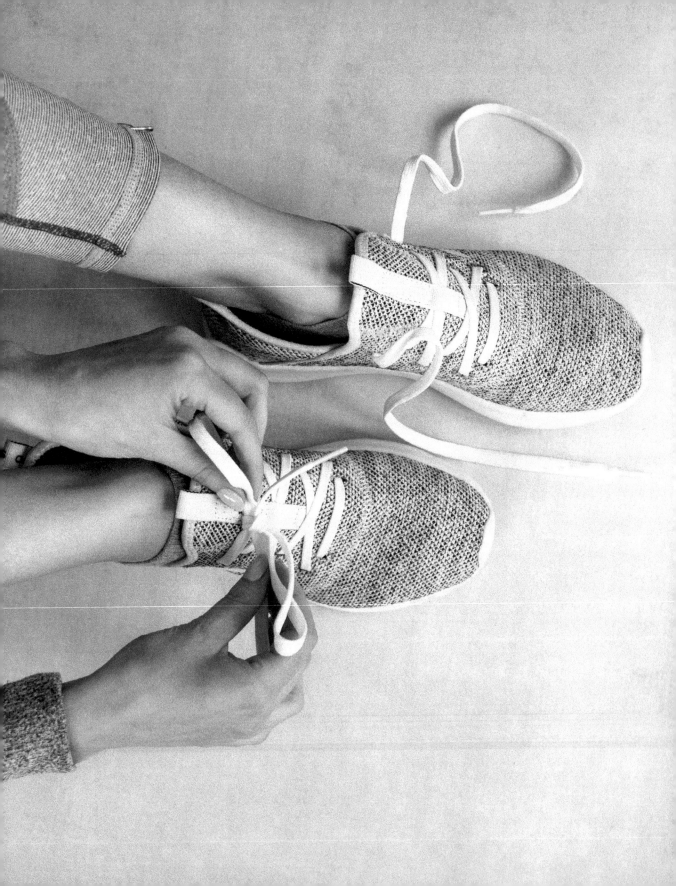

Chapter 2

Small Changes Make a Big Difference

Although there is no single cure for Lyme disease, it is entirely possible to reduce your symptoms and improve your overall health with diet and lifestyle changes. The human body is amazingly resilient; when we provide it with nutritious food, movement, and a healthy living environment, tremendous healing is possible!

Healthy and Realistic Lifestyle Changes

A clean environment

One of the greatest stumbling blocks to healing that I've observed among Lyme disease sufferers is the home environment. Living in an unhealthy environment significantly hinders healing from Lyme disease; conversely, cleaning up your environment can work wonders in accelerating your healing process.

If your present living environment is unhealthy, then the first step is to remove yourself from that environment. Possible factors that contribute to an unhealthy living environment include mold and mildew, environmental allergens, and volatile organic compounds (VOCs) released from items such as new carpet and paint. These contaminants aren't merely annoyances that cause you to sneeze or get a headache; research indicates that they can take a significant toll on your health.

Mold is a surprisingly common indoor contaminant that impairs overall health. It proliferates in water-damaged environments, growing on surfaces such as fiberboard, carpet, and ceiling tiles.

To keep your home free of mold and allergens, I recommend first investing in a high-quality air filtration system. An air filtration system will keep your air free of mold spores, dust, and other airborne allergens. You can choose either a whole-house system or individual air filter units for the room or rooms of your home where you spend the most time, such as your bedroom.

Investing in a water filtration system is also essential for supporting your health. Tap water may look clean, but it actually contains many industrial and agricultural contaminants that are harmful to our health. The Environmental Working Group, a nonprofit organization specializing in research on chemicals and human health, released a 2018 report demonstrating the presence of more than 250 contaminants in tap water. Although many of these contaminants are deemed perfectly legal according to the Safe Drinking Water Act, which is irrefutably outdated, they are well above levels found to be harmful in scientific studies. Contaminants identified in tap water samples from throughout the United States include the following:

Arsenic: Arsenic naturally occurs in the Earth's crust; it is released in large quantities by mining and is used as a pesticide. Arsenic is an established carcinogen.

Chromium-6: This industrial chemical was made notorious by the film *Erin Brockovich* and is linked to an increased risk of cancer.

Glyphosate: Glyphosate is an herbicide marketed as Roundup by Monsanto that is applied to crops and directly in people's yards to combat weeds. It is associated with an increased risk of cancer and disrupts the gut microbiome. Along with other pesticides, it may also increase the risk of autism.

Nitrate: Nitrate is a fertilizer chemical that ends up in drinking water due to agricultural and urban runoff. It is also associated with an increased risk of cancer.

Filtering your drinking and bathing water to remove contaminants will reduce your toxic burden, allowing your body to focus on fighting Lyme disease.

What to expect

Cleaning up your living and work spaces may not be the first thing that comes to mind when you think about Lyme disease recovery, though it can make a world of difference. You may be surprised to find that cleaning up indoor mold, with the help of a professional of course, helps you breathe easier, clears up chronic cough and sinus issues, and may even alleviate brain fog! Purifying your air may also help with respiratory issues and environmental allergies; filtering your water will reduce your exposure to harmful heavy metals and industrial and agricultural pollutants.

Perhaps most importantly, removing harmful contaminants from the air and water in your home will reduce your overall body burden of toxins. A decreased toxic burden will, in turn, take some of the strain off your detoxification pathways and immune system, improving the function of these systems and helping you gain ground against Lyme disease.

A toxin-free body

Unfortunately, toxins are ubiquitous in our modern-day environment. Toxins originate from industrial and agricultural processes and are found in our air, water, and food. Taking steps to filter your water and air, as mentioned earlier, will go a long way in terms of reducing your body burden of toxins. However, there are additional steps you can take to gently facilitate the removal of toxins from your body.

CILANTRO

Cilantro, a leafy herb with a distinct aroma, doesn't just add flavor to food; it is also a powerful agent for detoxifying heavy metals, including arsenic, cadmium, and lead. Do not underestimate cilantro's powerful healing properties. When consumed alone in high doses, cilantro may cause the body to redistribute heavy metals into sensitive tissues, such as the brain. To prevent this problem from occurring, cilantro should be consumed in conjunction with dietary fiber, which binds heavy metals and prevents their reabsorption into the systemic circulation.

LYME DISEASE AND MOLD ILLNESS

Mold illness, also known as Chronic Inflammatory Response Syndrome (CIRS), is a severe inflammatory disorder caused by exposure to environmental mold, mycotoxins, and other toxigenic organisms such as bacteria, endotoxins, and volatile organic compounds (VOCs). CIRS was first identified in 1997 by Dr. Ritchie Shoemaker, a family physician in the rural town of Pocomoke, Maryland, who found himself faced with a group of patients with an unusual set of symptoms, including gastrointestinal and neurological problems. He eventually traced the cause of his patients' illness to exposure to waterborne *Pfiesteria*, an organism associated with harmful algal blooms. Shoemaker soon realized that other biotoxins, particularly mold, could also cause significant illness, which led to coining of the term "mold illness."

The most common indoor molds capable of causing illness are *Cladosporium*, *Penicillium*, *Alternaria*, *Aspergillus*, and *Stachybotrys*. These molds produce a variety of by-products, including spores (the reproductive units of mold) and mycotoxins (toxic compounds that exert harmful effects throughout the body).

Mold and mycotoxins proliferate in water-damaged environments, where they enter the body via inhalation, ingestion, and skin exposure. Even though mold spores can precipitate allergies or asthma attacks, it is generally mycotoxins that are the most harmful. Shockingly, in the United States alone, 43 percent of buildings have current water damage and 85 percent have past water damage, indicating that exposure to mold and mycotoxins is far more common than one might expect! Mold illness is a growing concern due to climate change, which is creating a more hospitable environment for the growth of many molds, and due to the increasing virulence of mold strains as they've acquired resistance to common fungicides.

Mold and mycotoxins are also present in certain foods and can thereby be ingested. According to a 2016 study published in the scientific journal

Toxins, 25 percent of the world's crops, including grains, nuts, wine, spices, and coffee, are contaminated with mold and mycotoxins during harvesting, storage, and transportation. Mycotoxins may also accumulate in meat, eggs, and dairy products from animals fed mold-contaminated feed. Unfortunately, food processing doesn't neutralize mycotoxins, as most are thermally stable during boiling, baking, frying, roasting, and even pasteurization. People with mold illness may need to follow a low-mold diet to accelerate their recovery. A low-mold diet consists of fresh vegetables and fruits, raw nuts and seeds, grass-fed and organic meat and poultry, wild-caught seafood, and healthy fats such as olive oil and coconut oil. It eschews most fermented foods, such as cheese, sauerkraut, and alcoholic beverages, which have the potential to contain mold.

So, what does mold illness have to do with Lyme disease? Mold illness frequently accompanies Lyme disease because mold and mycotoxins impair immune function, making the body more susceptible to infections such as those caused by *Borrelia burgdorferi*. Mold and mycotoxins also cause intestinal dysbiosis, brain inflammation, hormonal imbalances, autoimmunity, and fatigue, exacerbating the symptoms of Lyme disease. If you have Lyme disease, continued exposure to mold and mycotoxins will seriously hinder your recovery process. Conversely, eliminating these toxins can have profound beneficial effects on your body.

To reduce your risk of mold illness, first make sure that your home and workplace are not water damaged and harboring mold. To determine whether mold is a problem in your environment, consider doing an Environmental Relative Moldiness Index (ERMI) test. The ERMI test identifies and quantifies bacteria and mold in your living environment and is considered the gold standard of mold-testing methods. DIY mold-testing kits are available from places such as Amazon and Home Depot, but I highly recommend spending the money for a professional ERMI test because DIY kits are notoriously inaccurate.

If your home is currently free of mold, keep it that way by maintaining an indoor humidity between 30 and 50 percent; ensuring proper ventilation for showers, laundry, and cooking areas; and making sure windows, roofs, and pipes are free of leaks.

BROCCOLI SPROUTS

Broccoli sprouts are young broccoli plants that look like alfalfa sprouts but have the sharp taste of radishes. They are rich in glucoraphanin, a precursor to the powerful phytochemical sulforaphane. When broccoli sprouts are chewed, an enzyme called myrosinase is released and transforms glucoraphanin into sulforaphane.

Sulforaphane is a potent detoxification agent. It activates phase II liver detoxification, in which toxic metabolites are converted into less toxic compounds that can then be excreted by the body. It normalizes liver enzymes and restores healthy liver function. Sulforaphane also stimulates the production of glutathione, a potent antioxidant that plays a crucial role in the body's defense against *Borrelia burgdorferi* infection. In addition to supporting detox, sulforaphane also supports immune function, reduces systemic inflammation, and eliminates harmful gastrointestinal microbes, all of which factor into the disease process in patients with Lyme disease.

Research suggests that you need to eat approximately 100 grams of broccoli sprouts per day to achieve therapeutic effects, including enhanced detoxification. To consume this quantity of broccoli sprouts without breaking the bank, I recommend growing them at home. All you need are organic broccoli seeds, a glass Mason jar, a sprouting lid, and a drainage stand, and you can continually reap the health benefits of this special vegetable!

DIETARY FIBER

Dietary fiber doesn't just keep your bowel habits "regular"; it also binds and facilitates the elimination of toxins from your body. Pectin, a type of soluble fiber found in apples, oranges, legumes, and oats, fortifies the intestinal barrier against harmful bacterial toxins and facilitates the excretion of lead, a harmful heavy metal. Modified citrus pectin, a unique form of pectin derived from the pith of citrus fruits, efficiently reduces the body burden of lead and may be a valuable addition to your detox protocol, alongside other pectin-rich foods.

SAUNA

A sauna isn't just a luxury to indulge in at the spa or sports club—it is actually a valuable detoxification tool that reduces your body's toxic burden by eliminating toxins through your sweat!

Sauna therapy is an ancient method of detoxifying the body that has been used by people around the world for thousands of years. In Finland, saunas are an integral part of the culture; historically, the sauna was considered the "poor man's pharmacy," a place to heal from a variety of maladies. In Russia, sauna (aka *banya*) was also used for regular cleansing and for purging the body of disease.

Today, scientific research has validated the ancestral uses of sauna therapy for healing. Studies show that sauna use enhances blood circulation and reduces systemic inflammation. It also induces profound sweating, ridding the body of toxins such as arsenic, cadmium, lead, mercury, organochlorine pesticides, flame retardants, and BPA.

Traditional cultures have long relied on steam and dry-heat saunas; however, these saunas must reach extremely high temperatures, typically between 150°F and 190°F, in order to warm the air sufficiently to induce sweating. These temperatures can be very uncomfortable for many people; fortunately, infrared saunas pose a lower-temperature, but equally beneficial, alternative. Infrared saunas use infrared thermal light to penetrate the skin, raising the body's core temperature and increasing blood flow without causing adverse effects such as light-headedness and high blood pressure. They operate at much lower temperatures than traditional saunas, typically between 110°F and 150°F, efficiently heating the body and promoting sweating without causing discomfort.

Are supplements useful for detoxification?

A healthy diet is the best source of vitamins and minerals for supporting detoxification, though supplements can provide an additional degree of support. Listed here are just a few supplements that are widely beneficial to patients with Lyme disease:

Magnesium: Magnesium is an essential cofactor for over 300 enzyme systems in the body, including many involved in detoxification. Unfortunately, according to a 2012 study published in *Nutrition Reviews*, nearly half of the U.S. population is magnesium deficient due to a low intake of magnesium-containing foods. Supplementing with around 300 mg of magnesium glycinate or magnesium orotate per day can boost your magnesium status and assist in detoxification.

Vitamin C: Vitamin C is a water-soluble vitamin that supports detoxification and regenerates endogenous antioxidants in the body, such as glutathione.

Glutathione: While your body produces glutathione (its "master antioxidant") naturally, glutathione stores are rapidly used up in the fight against *Borrelia burgdorferi*. Eating broccoli sprouts is one way to support your body's production of glutathione. However, you may also want to consider supplementing with liposomal glutathione, a highly bioavailable form of glutathione that detoxifies heavy metals, bacterial toxins, and mycotoxins, or with a glutathione precursor such as n-acetylcysteine or alpha-lipoic acid.

When selecting supplements, avoid those that contain ingredients such as titanium dioxide, artificial colorants, BHT, and sodium benzoate. These additives have been linked to many health problems, including DNA damage and liver toxicity.

What to expect

No matter whether you're in the early, mid, or chronic stages of Lyme disease, gently detoxifying your body will significantly support your recovery and help you achieve better health. However, keep in mind that in our modern-day world rife with environmental toxins, detoxification is not a short-term fix; rather, it is a set of lifestyle changes that must be consistently practiced if you want to experience long-term benefits. With consistent use of the detoxification strategies mentioned here, you may notice a clearer mind, increased energy, decreased pain and inflammation, improved digestive system function, and more restful sleep.

A note on dental work: *Dental work can significantly increase your toxic load, if done incorrectly. Amalgam fillings are known to release mercury vapors and, if removed incorrectly, can cause mercury toxicity. Root canals and tooth removals can lead to cavitations and infections, further increasing your bacterial toxic load. This is a loaded topic that could fill an entire book, so we will not be able to delve into it here. If you have fillings or other dental issues, I recommend checking out the website of the International Academy of Biological Dentistry & Medicine to find a dentist in your area familiar with the safe removal of fillings and treatment of dental infections, so that you can decide the best course of treatment.*

Gentle exercise

It can be difficult to drum up the motivation to exercise when you're struggling with the fatigue, lethargy, and joint discomfort associated with Lyme disease. However, gentle exercise is truly crucial for promoting recovery from Lyme disease for several reasons:

Exercise activates the lymphatic system, your body's system for removing waste products from your cells and regulating immunity. It is a complex network composed of vessels, ducts, lymph nodes, and your spleen, thymus, adenoids, and tonsils.

INTERMITTENT FASTING:
PROVEN METHOD OR PASSING TREND?

Intermittent fasting, an eating strategy in which you eat meals within a specific time period each day and fast the rest of the time, has taken the wellness world by storm. Despite its recent popularity, intermittent fasting is far from just a passing trend! Humans have fasted intermittently for much of history due to variations in food availability. Many scientists believe that our evolutionary heritage has programmed us to derive health benefits from fasting. A rapidly growing body of research supports this theory, and several lines of research indicate intermittent fasting may be particularly beneficial for patients with Lyme disease:

- Intermittent fasting activates autophagy, the process by which your cells clean out old, damaged components. Research indicates that autophagy reduces *B. burgdorferi*–induced inflammation and that induction of autophagy may promote recovery from Lyme disease.

- It alleviates cognitive dysfunction caused by brain inflammation, a pervasive problem in sufferers of Lyme disease.

- It supports the growth of beneficial gut bacteria. This effect may benefit patients with Lyme disease who've been on repeated rounds of antibiotics and need to regenerate a healthy gut microbiota.

If you are interested in trying intermittent fasting, I recommend beginning by restricting your meals to an 8- to 10-hour time window each day. The remaining 14 to 16 hours of the day and night should be spent in a fasting state. For example, if you eat dinner at 6 p.m., refrain from eating again until 8 a.m. or 10 a.m. the next day; research suggests that time frame is the most effective for achieving the health benefits of intermittent fasting.

Although intermittent fasting can benefit many patients with Lyme disease, there is an important caveat: If you are underweight or tend to undereat, I advise against intermittent fasting because it may further reduce your appetite and promote weight loss. Pregnant and breastfeeding women should also avoid fasting since they require a constant supply of nutrients to support their baby's growth and development.

Unlike the circulatory system, the lymphatic system does not have its own pump (the heart) to promote fluid circulation and drainage. Instead, it relies on skeletal muscle movement to transport and filter lymph fluid. If you remain sedentary, your lymphatic system will become stagnant, causing a buildup of immune cells, bacterial waste products, and toxins in your tissues. Gentle exercise, on the other hand, pumps lymphatic fluid throughout your body, cleansing your body of the waste products generated as your body works to eradicate Lyme disease.

Exercise boosts immune function. Regular exercise is good for your whole body, promoting cardiovascular health, lowering blood pressure, and helping to control body weight—and when your body is healthier, your immune system is healthier, too. More specifically, exercise improves circulation throughout your body, which helps the antibodies, cells, chemicals, and proteins that make up the immune system move freely to locate and destroy bacteria and viruses.

Exercise boosts brain function. Brain inflammation and cognitive dysfunction are common symptoms of Lyme disease, but they can be alleviated with regular exercise! Exercise promotes the endogenous release of brain-derived neurotrophic factor (BDNF), a neuroprotective compound that has anti-inflammatory effects on the brain. Importantly, you don't need to push yourself extremely hard to get the exercise-induced benefits of BDNF; aerobic exercise at a moderate heart rate (60 percent of your heart rate reserve—the difference between resting heart rate and maximum heart rate) significantly increases BDNF. You can achieve this heart rate through gentle jogging or cycling.

Exercise stimulates feel-good neurotransmitters. Depression and anxiety are common comorbidities with Lyme disease. Exercise is a valuable, drug-free means of ameliorating these conditions because it promotes the release of dopamine, norepinephrine, and serotonin, brain chemicals that play crucial roles in regulating mood.

Top five at-home exercises for joint pain management

Exercise should be a central component of any Lyme disease treatment plan. However, if you are dealing with significant joint pain, I recommend beginning with exercises specifically intended for joint pain management. The following exercises are helpful for reducing pain in the knees, lower back, and neck.

Leg lifts: Leg lifts improve stability and balance and strengthen your legs, reducing impact on your knees. To perform a leg lift, first stand against a wall. Raise your right or left leg to the side, keeping your toe pointing forward or slightly in. Lower the leg. Repeat 15 to 20 times on each side. *Add a resistance band to make this exercise more challenging.*

Hamstring stretch: If you spend much of your day sitting, this exercise is a must! It improves your range of motion and will reduce your risk of pain and injuries from exercise. To perform the exercise, lie on your back and loop a yoga strap or scarf over one foot. Use the strap or scarf to pull your leg straight up. Hold for 20 seconds and lower. Repeat twice on each leg.

Partial crunches: Partial crunches strengthen your back and abdominal muscles to help reduce lower back pain. Lie with your knees bent and feet flat on the floor. Tighten your abdominal muscles and raise your shoulders off the floor. Hold for a second, then lower back down. Repeat 8 to 12 times.

Wall sits: Wall sits allow you to experience the benefits of a squat without stressing your back. Stand 10 to 12 inches from a wall and lean back until your back is flat against the wall. Slide down, bending your knees and pressing your lower back against the wall. Hold for 10 seconds and slowly slide back up the wall. Repeat 8 to 12 times.

Neck release: Neck pain is common in patients with Lyme disease. To release your neck, start with your head squarely over your shoulders and your back straight. Lower your chin to your chest and hold for 30 seconds. Lift your head back up and tip it backward, with your chin toward the ceiling. Repeat three to four times.

How to exercise when you are low on energy

Deciding whether to exercise when you're feeling low on energy can be a conundrum. On the one hand, exercising when your body is truly struggling to stay afloat can drain your energy reserves. However, in other cases, low energy can be boosted by exercise.

If you are running a fever or just had an operation, give your body permission to skip exercise; pushing yourself in these situations could make you feel much worse or impair your recovery.

If you tend to struggle more with the mental aspect of exercising, write a motivational reminder about exercise on a Post-it and stick it in a location where you will see it daily. For example, the reminder could say something like "Exercise creates energy!"

WAYS TO PROTECT YOUR JOINTS

When performing exercises, start slowly. Gradually increase the number of sets and reps for each exercise. If you feel that an exercise is worsening your pain, listen to your body's signals and stop.

Incorporate movement into daily life. Even if you have a regular exercise routine, sitting all day can counteract its benefits. If you have a highly sedentary job or lifestyle, try to take walking and standing breaks throughout the day. In my case, investing in a standing desk has made a world of difference in how much movement I fit in every day, and I highly recommend buying one if your job requires extended periods of sitting.

Pay attention to proper body mechanics. Whichever exercises you choose to do, make sure you are using proper form because poor form can increase your risk of injury.

How to treat your body after exercise

To enhance your post-exercise recovery, try the following strategies:

Replace lost fluids: Drink plenty of filtered water after your exercise session. Consider mixing in a natural electrolyte powder that is free of artificial colors, flavors, and added sugars.

Stretch: Stretching post-exercise will help your muscles recover faster.

Use a foam roller: A foam roller is an inexpensive but invaluable tool for reducing muscle stiffness and pain and improving mobility.

Get a massage: Massage is an excellent way to promote recovery from exercise. It has the side benefits of reducing stress and boosting immune function! There are many types of massage out there, including deep tissue and Thai massage, Shiatsu, and Rolfing; explore a couple different techniques to find the best one for your needs.

Take an Epsom salt bath: Epsom salts contain a form of magnesium that is readily absorbed through the skin and has muscle-relaxant effects. To take an Epsom

EXERCISE WITHOUT JOINING A GYM

You do not need an expensive gym membership to maintain an exercise routine. There are many exercises that you can do in the comfort of your own home or outdoors in nature.

Yoga encompasses many exercises that are beneficial for relieving joint pain. Find an instructional yoga video with a focus on restorative poses and practice at least three to four days a week. Avoid more vigorous types of yoga, such as Vinyasa and Bikram yoga, as these may exacerbate joint pain.

Tai Chi is a Chinese mind-body exercise therapy that is an effective adjunct treatment for chronic pain conditions. Try an instructional Tai Chi video at home, such as *Tai Chi for Beginners*, available on Amazon.

Rubber resistance bands are a great, inexpensive tool for strengthening your muscles. Try simple exercises such as lateral lunges, lateral leg raises, and biceps curls with a resistance band for a convenient workout.

Range-of-motion (ROM) exercises help maintain mobility and flexibility and improve joint function. A physical therapist can help you determine which ROM exercises may be most beneficial for you.

Walking—yes, plain old walking—can improve joint pain! Many of us lead quite sedentary lives; in fact, research indicates that one in four American adults sits for over eight hours a day! Long periods of uninterrupted sitting cause joint, muscle, and tendon pain and stiffness. Taking a daily 30-minute walk over your lunch break or after work can do wonders for relieving pain and stiffness.

salt bath, first fill your tub with hot water. Next, add two cups of Epsom salt to the bathtub and let it dissolve. Soak in the tub for at least 10 minutes to get the full benefits of the Epsom salts.

Meditation

Chronic stress wreaks havoc on the immune system and makes it harder for the body to recover from infectious illnesses. If you really want to kick Lyme disease to the curb, engaging in a daily stress-reduction practice is essential. Meditation is a time-honored and scientifically proven strategy for reducing stress that also offers many downstream health benefits applicable to Lyme patients.

So, what are the benefits of meditation for Lyme disease patients? It turns out that there are quite a few, including improved immune function, reduced inflammation, better mental health and brain health, pain relief, and improved sleep.

IMPROVES IMMUNE FUNCTION

Meditation has been found to alter the expression of genes that regulate immunity, reducing unproductive inflammatory responses and enabling immune cells to better respond to pathogens such as *Borrelia burgdorferi*.

REDUCES INFLAMMATION

Chronic inflammation is a characteristic feature of Lyme disease. In fact, it is believed to be the common underlying cause of the fatigue, cognitive dysfunction, and pain associated with the disease. Fortunately, meditation can help diminish that inflammation! Research indicates that meditation reduces levels of circulating inflammatory proteins.

SUPPORTS MENTAL HEALTH

Unfortunately, anxiety and depression are common comorbidities in Lyme disease, due to the significant emotional toll of the disease. However, studies have found that engaging in just 30 minutes of meditation a day significantly alleviates anxiety and depression. An improved mental outlook can, in turn, facilitate recovery from illness.

BOOSTS BRAIN HEALTH

Scientific studies have shown that meditation boosts neuroplasticity, the process by which the brain reorganizes itself and forms new neural connections in response to injury or changes in one's environment. Neuroplasticity failure (the inability to successfully "rewire" neural connections) is associated with cognitive dysfunction and an increased risk of neurodegenerative diseases such as Alzheimer's disease. Strategies that support neuroplasticity, such as meditation, will therefore help support optimal brain health over the long term.

Meditation can reduce chronic pain, a characteristic feature of Lyme disease, by decreasing circulating levels of pro-inflammatory cytokines. It can also alter neural pathways in the brain that process pain signals, leading to an attenuation of physical pain.

IMPROVES SLEEP

Sleep is essential for recovering from any illness, including Lyme disease. Research indicates that meditation improves sleep. An eight-week meditation program has been found to decrease sleep disturbances, eliminate insomnia, and improve sleep quality, including the duration and depth of sleep.

So what's the best way to get started with meditation? Many people are hesitant to begin a meditation practice because they are overwhelmed by the available options, including online meditation programs, books, and apps. I recommend that meditation newbies start by using a convenient, free app such as Headspace, Calm, or Waking Up. These apps offer helpful guided meditations, with many averaging just a few minutes in length, making meditation an easy addition to your daily routine. Once you've committed to a consistent meditation practice—I typically recommend trying to meditate twice a day, once in the morning and once before bed—you may want to try other options such as a meditation class.

Insider Tip

ACUPUNCTURE FOR PAIN RELIEF

If you are plagued with chronic pain, acupuncture is one alternative pain relief solution you'll want to try! Acupuncture, an ancient Chinese practice in which fine needles are inserted into specific points on the body, can have both immediate and long-term analgesic effects. In several studies, acupuncture has been found more effective for immediate pain relief than analgesic drug injections! It is effective for musculoskeletal, headache, and arthritic pain, and has no side effects.

Though acupuncture is a very low-risk approach, it typically is not covered by health insurance. If you are interested in trying acupuncture, ask your medical provider for the name of a recommended certified practitioner.

Importantly, meditation isn't just limited to sitting quietly, eyes closed, in a chair. Taking a walk outdoors in a beautiful natural area, practicing yoga, and even engaging in a beloved hobby can be considered forms of meditation, as long as they are done with mindful awareness and without extraneous distractions.

Sleep

Sleep is a frequently overlooked but crucial determinant of our health status. In fact, it is so important that I consider it a "make-or-break" factor in the Lyme disease recovery process.

How does your body respond when you don't get enough sleep?

The human body does not respond well to sleep deprivation. Studies have shown that short sleep duration, defined as sleeping less than seven to eight hours a night, impairs immune function (and thus your ability to fight *B. burgdorferi*), lowers pain tolerance, increases inflammation, and impairs insulin sensitivity and metabolic function. In other words, sleep deprivation leaves you at an increased risk of infection, inflamed, in pain, and suffering from dramatic blood sugar swings.

Sleep disruption, which refers to frequent sleep interruptions despite a potentially normal sleep duration, is also harmful to our health. In a 2017 study published in *Nature and Science of Sleep*, scientists concluded that sleep disruption increases pain; promotes depression, anxiety, and cognitive dysfunction; and reduces immune function. These problems spell trouble for patients with Lyme disease, who are already struggling with chronic pain, mental health issues, brain dysfunction, and impaired immunity.

How does your body respond when you do get enough sleep?

Sufficient sleep is essential for helping the body heal from sickness and injury. Getting plenty of sleep helps your body boost immune function, reduce pain and inflammation, and improve cognitive function.

Good habits that induce quality sleep

There are several steps you can take to improve your sleep each night:

Sleep in a completely dark room. Artificial light exposure disrupts the body's production of melatonin, a crucial sleep-inducing hormone, and can impair the sleep cycle. Remove night-lights and other light-emitting devices from your bedroom and invest in some room-darkening shades to prevent light from streetlamps and other buildings from entering your room.

Reduce the temperature of your bedroom. Lowering the ambient temperature of your bedroom at night can help induce sleep. According to scientific studies, 67°F is the temperature most effective for inducing sleep.

Reduce blue light exposure before bed. Blue light, a type of light emitted from digital devices such as smartphones, tablets, computer screens, television, and fluorescent and LED lights, disrupts your body's production of melatonin. This results in difficulty getting to sleep and reduced sleep quality. To reduce your blue light exposure in the evening, put your cellphone in "nighttime" mode, download the f.lux or Iris apps for your computer, and wear blue-light-blocking glasses for at least an hour before heading to bed.

Log off social media at least one hour before bed. Social media use tends to induce a sympathetic nervous system response (aka "fight-or-flight" mode), which is a state of mind you do not want to be in right before bed! Instead of scrolling through Instagram or Facebook before you hit the sack, meditate, read a book, or write in a journal. These activities will calm your nervous system and promote quality sleep.

What to expect

Improving your sleep habits will boost your health, whether you are in the early, mid, or late stages of Lyme disease. Committing to getting seven to eight hours of sleep per night, as well as practicing good sleep hygiene before bed, will leave you feeling more rested and energetic in the morning. It may also reduce inflammation and pain, improve your cognitive function, and leave you feeling more positive! Sleep may be an afterthought for much of our population, but given the enormous health implications of sleep loss, you should make it a top priority in your life.

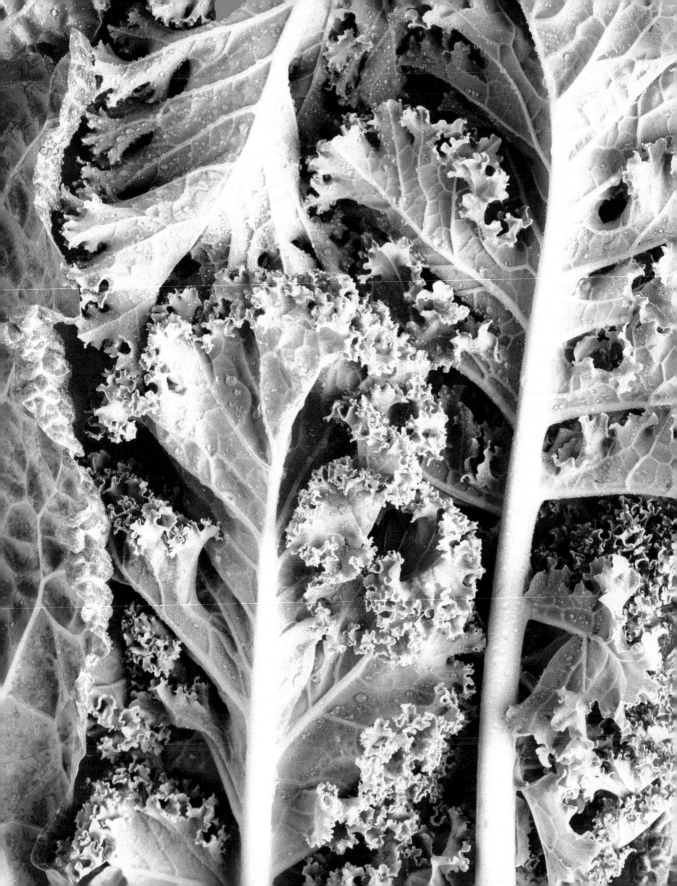

Chapter **3**

The Detox Diet

What are the best foods to eat and avoid to promote
detoxification and alleviate the inflammation, pain, cognitive
dysfunction, and fatigue associated with Lyme disease? In this
chapter, we will cover all the basics you need to know to implement
a diet that will reduce inflammation, help your body eliminate
toxins, and ease your Lyme disease symptoms.

Before you dive into this diet, you should know that many
people with Lyme disease must avoid gluten to reduce inflammation, optimize gut health, and ease symptoms. Gluten is found in
wheat, barley, rye, and numerous processed and packaged foods.
Some may be able to tolerate small amounts of gluten-containing
grains on occasion if those grains are organic, ancient, or, as in the
case of sourdough bread, fermented. The fermentation process used
to create sourdough increases the solubility of gluten proteins by
breaking down their disulfide bonds. That being said, gluten should
not be a frequent part of the diet and complete avoidance may produce the best results for Lyme patients.

Benefits of Detox

Foods rich in antioxidants can reduce inflammation

Some of the best foods you can eat to support your recovery from Lyme disease are those rich in antioxidants. Antioxidant-rich foods combat inflammation via several mechanisms.

- Some antioxidant nutrients, such as vitamins C and E, reduce inflammation by directly scavenging free radicals—atoms with unpaired electrons that are highly reactive and damage DNA, proteins, and tissues in the body. Vitamins C and E quench free radicals by donating electrons to the radicals, satisfying the radicals, "desire" for more electrons and thereby reducing their reactivity.

- Some antioxidant nutrients, particularly phytochemicals found in plant foods, reduce inflammation by activating the body's own antioxidant systems. These phytochemicals actually induce a mild stress response in the body, referred to as a "hormetic effect." This response is an upregulation of antioxidant systems. One such system, the Nrf2 system, ultimately triggers the production of glutathione, your body's "master antioxidant."

Lyme disease is essentially an inflammatory disease, so any dietary approach to treating the disease should focus heavily on the consumption of antioxidant-rich foods. Consuming high-antioxidant foods such as berries, cruciferous vegetables, and olive oil can significantly relieve symptoms of Lyme disease that are rooted in inflammation, such as brain fog, fatigue, and joint pain.

Healthy food can ease symptoms

Healthy food in moderation combined with a healthy lifestyle will not cure symptoms but certainly will work to ease them.

Unfortunately, there is no single food that will erase your Lyme disease symptoms. However, eating a nutrient-dense, anti-inflammatory diet *does* create a strong foundation for optimal health. By providing your body with all the nutrients it needs to support optimal immune function, avoid inflammation, and assist in detoxification, a healthy diet can significantly alleviate symptoms of Lyme disease and help you regain your health.

Just like healthy foods can promote recovery from Lyme disease, unhealthy foods (especially refined carbohydrates, industrial seed oils, and food additives) can hinder it.

Importantly, a healthy diet works best in conjunction with healthy lifestyle changes. Many of the lifestyle changes mentioned in chapter 2, including detox strategies, intermittent fasting, a consistent exercise routine, meditation, and sleep, work synergistically with dietary changes to facilitate recovery from Lyme disease and promote optimal long-term health.

Detox to restore the gut

In addition to reducing inflammation, a successful dietary approach to treating Lyme disease should also actively work to restore optimal gut health. Almost 70 percent of the human immune system resides in the gut; your immune system regulates your response to *Borrelia burgdorferi*, and immune dysfunction resulting in chronic inflammation is at the root of chronic Lyme disease. Therefore, if you want to improve your immune function to beat Lyme disease, then gut health should be a priority!

There are two main dietary steps you can take to restore your gut health and optimize your immune function:

1. **Banish inflammatory foods that are compromising your gut health.** For many, the consumption of gluten precipitates an inflammatory response in the gut, necessitating the removal of gluten-containing foods. Consider a trial elimination of gluten for nine weeks to see if any of your symptoms subside; alternately, you can test for gluten sensitivity with the help of a functional medicine doctor or nutritionist. I recommend Cyrex Laboratories' celiac and gluten sensitivity panel for testing for gluten sensitivity. You may also need to remove dairy foods if they contribute to inflammation in your body. You can test for dairy sensitivity using an IgE/IgG food sensitivity test. Some people may also benefit from doing a comprehensive elimination diet, in which they remove foods most commonly known to cause an inflammatory response.

2. **Restore the integrity of your gut lining with gut-healing and probiotic-containing foods.** Collagen and gelatin powder from grass-fed cows contain amino acids that help repair the intestinal lining. Fermented foods such as kimchi, coconut or almond milk yogurt, and kombucha contain probiotics that replenish the gut microbiota. A healthy gut microbiota, in turn, reduces intestinal inflammation and helps restore a healthy gut lining.

Dietary Rules and Guidelines

Foods to enjoy freely

On the Detox Diet, there are many foods that you can enjoy freely.

NONSTARCHY VEGETABLES

Nonstarchy vegetables are rich in insoluble fiber, which keeps food moving through your digestive tract, B vitamins, vitamin C, vitamin K_1, and anti-inflammatory phyto-nutrients that support immune, gut, and brain function.

Aim for *at least* 3 to 4 servings a day of nonstarchy vegetables. Choose from the following:

- Asparagus
- Bok choy
- Broccoli
- Brussels sprouts
- Carrots
- Cauliflower
- Green beans
- Leafy greens (spinach, Swiss chard, kale, collard greens, butter lettuce, romaine lettuce)
- Leeks
- Onion
- Peppers
- Radishes
- Shallots
- Summer squash
- Tomatoes

I strongly recommend buying seasonal and organic produce as much as possible to limit your exposure to pesticides. Please refer to The Dirty Dozen and the Clean Fifteen™ appendix (see page 127) to learn which vegetables (and fruits) you should buy organic and which are safe to buy conventional.

PROTEIN

Aim to eat a serving of protein with each meal; this will help stabilize your blood sugar throughout the day, support tissue repair, and provide your body with the amino acids it needs to support detoxification and optimal immune function.

Animal proteins:

- Beef
- Bison
- Chicken
- Collagen powder from pastured cows (this is a great food for joint support)

- Eggs
- Lamb
- Pork
- Turkey
- Wild game (elk, wild boar)
- Wild-caught seafood and shellfish

Try to choose organic, grass-fed, and pastured animal proteins as much as possible.

Vegetable proteins:

- Buckwheat
- Chickpeas
- Lentils
- Organic tempeh
- Organic tofu
- Peanut butter
- Quinoa
- Sprouted grain bread

It is important to realize that vegetarian and vegan proteins also tend to be high in carbohydrates, which, as we will dive into shortly, can cause some problems when consumed in large quantities. Furthermore, to obtain the full spectrum of amino acids your body needs to support detoxification and immune function, you'll need to combine vegetable proteins, such as lentils and quinoa. If you choose to eat soy products, such as tofu and tempeh, choose organic because non-organic soy is typically genetically modified.

HEALTHY FATS

Healthy fats reduce inflammation and support cognitive function and should therefore comprise a significant portion of your diet. Wild-caught seafood is the best dietary source of the omega-3 fatty acids EPA and DHA, which are crucial for regulating inflammatory balance and brain function. Though you can obtain a precursor to DHA and EPA, called alpha-linolenic acid (ALA), from plant foods such as chia seeds and flaxseed, the conversion of ALA to DHA and EPA is relatively inefficient. As a result, consuming wild-caught seafood such as salmon, mackerel, and sardines is highly recommended to individuals recovering from Lyme disease.

Other healthy fats to include are the following:

- Avocado oil
- Avocados
- Chia seeds
- Coconut oil
- Freshly ground flaxseed
- Hemp seeds
- Nuts and nut butter (almonds, macadamia nuts, walnuts, hazelnuts, cashews)
- Olive oil

Use heat-stable coconut oil and avocado oil for cooking. Olive oil should only be used for sautéing or topping already cooked foods because its fatty acids are more delicate and susceptible to damage from heat and light. Nut and seed oils (such as walnut oil and flax oil) should never be heated due to their high propensity to turn rancid when heated.

Foods to eat in moderation

On the Detox Diet, the foods that I recommend eating in moderation are starchy carbohydrates and whole fruits.

Starchy carbohydrates, found in foods such as root vegetables, grains, and legumes, have multiple health benefits. The first benefit is that they provide your body with glucose for energy production! A second benefit is that they contain prebiotic fiber, a type of dietary fiber that acts as food for the beneficial bacteria in your gut. Sweet potatoes, oats, and chickpeas are just a few examples of starchy carbohydrates rich in prebiotic fiber. Finally, starchy carbohydrates are good sources of potassium, magnesium, selenium, and several B vitamins.

Choose from the following starchy carbohydrates:

- Beets
- Cassava
- Celeriac
- Gluten-free whole grains (quinoa, buckwheat, millet, sorghum)
- Legumes (chickpeas, lentils, black beans, kidney beans, white beans)
- Plantains
- Rutabaga
- Sweet potatoes
- Turnips
- Whole grains
- Winter squash (butternut, acorn, delicata)

Whole fruits also have many health benefits. They are rich in phytonutrients that reduce inflammation and promote the establishment of a healthy gut microbiota. They are also excellent sources of potassium, vitamin C, and fiber. Choose from the following fruits:

- Apples
- Berries (blueberries, raspberries, blackberries, strawberries, currants)
- Citrus fruits (oranges, grapefruit, lemon, lime)
- Figs
- Nectarines
- Papaya
- Peaches
- Pears
- Pineapple

Starchy carbohydrates and whole fruits certainly have health benefits, but I recommend moderating your consumption of them for two main reasons:

A high carbohydrate intake can cause hyperglycemia and blood sugar fluctuations. When the body is inflamed by factors such as chronic infection, it may become less sensitive to insulin, the hormone that shuttles glucose from the bloodstream into cells for energy production. This condition, referred to as insulin resistance, causes blood sugar levels to rise. High blood sugar, or hyperglycemia, has been found to impair the body's ability to clear *Borrelia burgdorferi*. If you want to enhance your body's ability to fight off Lyme disease, then improving your blood sugar control by moderating your carbohydrate intake is crucial.

A high carbohydrate intake may exacerbate gut dysbiosis. Intestinal dysbiosis, an imbalance between good and bad microbes in the gut, is common in patients with Lyme disease. A high intake of starchy carbs can promote the growth of opportunistic and pathogenic bacteria, worsening dysbiosis.

Finding the right intake of carbohydrates for your needs may take some trial and error. Start by having one to two servings of starchy carbohydrates and one to two servings of fruit per day; if this feels good to you, stick with it. If not, you may need to reduce or increase your intake, depending on your activity level, metabolism, and current state of gut health.

Foods to restrict or avoid

REFINED CARBOHYDRATES

A high intake of refined carbohydrates from bread, pasta, cakes, cookies, ice cream, and candy causes blood sugar fluctuations and hyperglycemia, and disrupts the gut microbiota. Replace these foods with nonstarchy vegetables and moderate amounts of starchy, nutrient-dense carbohydrates and whole fruits, as mentioned previously.

INDUSTRIAL SEED OILS

Industrial seed oils are the highly processed oils expressed from canola, corn, cottonseed, soybean, and safflower seeds. These oils were only introduced to the human diet in the early 1900s, when a surplus of these commodity crops led several sly manufacturers to begin advertising the oils—previously used only for industrial purposes—as "heart-healthy" alternatives to animal fat. Sadly, though they did catch on, those health claims were pure fiction.

Industrial seed oils are high in omega-6 fatty acids. A high intake of omega-6 at the expense of omega-3 fatty acids (which many Americans are deficient in) creates a pro-inflammatory state in the body, which is not conducive to healing from Lyme disease.

Industrial seed oils are processed using harmful additives such as BHA, BHT, and TBHQ. Studies have shown that consumption of these additives disrupts hormones, impairs immune function, and may even promote allergies.

Due to their chemical structure, industrial seed oils are highly unstable and oxidize rapidly in response to light and heat. These processes create highly inflammatory and toxic trans fats. The consumption of trans fats triggers a chain reaction of free radical damage and inflammation in the body.

Industrial seed oils are frequently derived from genetically modified (GM) crops. These crops may be harmful to the gut microbiota and immune system.

DAIRY

The proteins in dairy are highly inflammatory for many people. Furthermore, non-organic dairy is a source of artificial hormones and pesticide residues. If you do choose to eat dairy, buy only hormone- and antibiotic-free, organic, and grass-fed products. Fermented dairy, such as yogurt and kefir, is best because it provides probiotics.

ARTIFICIAL SWEETENERS

A growing body of research indicates that artificial sweeteners disrupt the gut microbiota and compromise brain function. Avoid all artificial sweeteners, including aspartame (NutraSweet, Equal), saccharin (Sweet'N Low), sucralose (Splenda), and acesulfame potassium (Sweet One) and any foods that contain these sweeteners. For a healthy noncaloric sweetener, choose stevia or monk fruit extract.

FARMED SEAFOOD

Farmed seafood is high in environmental toxins, such as PCBs and dioxin. It is also low in nutrients compared to wild-caught seafood.

ARTIFICIAL COLORANTS AND PRESERVATIVES

Artificial colorants and preservatives are linked to gut inflammation and brain and immune dysfunction. The top additives to avoid are MSG, FD&C colors (such as Blue #1 and #2), sodium sulfite, sodium nitrate, sulfur dioxide, and potassium bromate.

Foods to Enjoy

ALMONDS

EXAMPLES

- Grab a handful with an apple for a quick snack
- Use to top oatmeal or "noatmeal"
- Add to fruit and nut bars or trail mix

BENEFITS

- Great source of vitamin E, a fat-soluble vitamin with antioxidant properties
- Good source of calcium (~95 mg per ¼-cup serving) for those on a dairy-free diet

BLUEBERRIES

EXAMPLES

- Add to a smoothie, mix with coconut or almond milk yogurt, or just eat plain

BENEFITS

- Contain polyphenols with antioxidant and anti-inflammatory effects. According to a 2014 study published in *Neural Regeneration Research*, blueberries can decrease neuroinflammation and enhance brain function.
- Support the establishment of an anti-inflammatory gut microbiota, which can improve systemic inflammation

CACAO/DARK CHOCOLATE

EXAMPLES

- Add cacao to smoothies or have a few squares of dark chocolate for dessert. Aim for dark chocolate with a 75% or higher cacao content.

BENEFITS

- Cacao and cocoa, the dried and fully fermented cacao seed, contain antioxidant compounds that have been shown to reduce neuroinflammation and enhance cognition, attention, and memory
- Can help induce the release of nitric oxide, improving blood flow and protecting the cardiovascular system
- May help enhance the gut immune system and promote the growth of an anti-inflammatory gut microbiota

Foods to Enjoy

CINNAMON

EXAMPLES

- Top a baked apple or pear with coconut cream and cinnamon for a delicious dessert
- Add to oatmeal for a cozy, comforting breakfast

BENEFITS

- Contains oils that can act as antibacterial agents against *Borrelia burgdorferi*
- May support healthy blood sugar control

COCONUT OIL

EXAMPLES

- Use for roasting vegetables, cooking eggs, and in baking
- Add to smoothies, oatmeal, or "noatmeal" for a dose of healthy, satiating fat

BENEFITS

- Contains fatty acids that have demonstrated antimicrobial activity against *C. difficile, Candida albicans*, intestinal parasites, and oral pathogens without harming beneficial bacteria
- Contains medium-chain triglycerides (MCTs) that can help increase blood ketone levels to support cognitive function

CRUCIFEROUS VEGETABLES
(broccoli, broccoli sprouts, cauliflower, kale, radishes, rutabaga)

EXAMPLES

- Sauté broccoli, cauliflower, and kale lightly in olive oil or avocado oil
- Massage kale with olive oil, then add other chopped vegetables and pumpkin seeds to make a salad
- Enjoy raw radishes with dip, such as hummus. You can make delicious veggie "noodles" with rutabaga and a spiralizer
- Eat broccoli sprouts raw in a sandwich/wrap or mixed into a salad

BENEFITS

- Contain fiber, vitamins C and K_1, carotenoids, and folate
- Broccoli sprouts contain a large amount of glucoraphanin, the precursor to sulforaphane. Sulforaphane stimulates glutathione production, enhancing your body's antioxidant defenses.

Foods to Enjoy

EGGS

EXAMPLES	BENEFITS
• Eat scrambled or hardboiled, or use to make "egg muffins" for breakfast	• The best dietary source of choline, a nutrient that has been shown to support liver detoxification and brain function

FERMENTED FOODS

EXAMPLES	BENEFITS
• Try kimchi, coconut or almond milk yogurt and kefir, and kombucha	• Rich in probiotics, which have been shown to support a healthy gut microbiota, immune system, and brain function

GARLIC AND ONIONS

EXAMPLES	BENEFITS
• Add to stir-fries, omelets and "egg muffins," soups, and stews	• Essential oils from garlic have been shown to kill persistent *Borrelia burgdorferi* • Onions contain inulin, a prebiotic fiber that supports the growth of beneficial gut bacteria

GRASS-FED BEEF

EXAMPLES	BENEFITS
• Make burgers or meatballs; add to stir-fries and stews	• Rich in highly bioavailable heme iron, vitamin B_{12}, omega-3 fatty acids, carotenoids, and antioxidants

OATS

EXAMPLES	BENEFITS
• Mix with coconut or almond milk, fruit, and almond butter for a satisfying breakfast • Make homemade granola or granola bars	• Good source of prebiotic fiber for feeding beneficial gut bacteria

Foods to Enjoy

OLIVE OIL

EXAMPLES	BENEFITS
• Drizzle on salads or cooked vegetables • Do not use for high-heat cooking (frying, roasting) because high heat reduces the antioxidant content of olive oil	• Supports brain health • Reduces inflammation • Has been shown to have antimicrobial and antiviral effects

WALNUTS

EXAMPLES	BENEFITS
• Add to fruit and nut bars, use to top salads, or eat plain	• Contain anti-inflammatory polyphenols and fatty acids

WILD-CAUGHT SALMON

EXAMPLES	BENEFITS
• Sauté or bake in the oven	• One of the best dietary sources of EPA and DHA, two omega-3 fatty acids that are crucial for brain health and reducing inflammation

Foods to Avoid

ARTIFICIAL SWEETENERS

EXAMPLES	REASON TO AVOID
• Diet soda, diet foods, saccharin, acesulfame, aspartame, neotame, Sucralose	• Have been shown to alter the gut microbiota, reducing levels of beneficial gut bacteria and promoting the growth of pathogens

CONVENTIONALLY GROWN FRUITS AND VEGETABLES ON THE "DIRTY DOZEN" LIST
(these should only be bought organic)

EXAMPLES	REASON TO AVOID
• Strawberries, spinach, kale, nectarines, apples, grapes, peaches, cherries, pears, tomatoes, celery, potatoes	• These fruits and vegetables are high in pesticides that are harmful to gut microbes, the reproductive system, and the brain • *Note: If you cannot afford to buy these items organic, check out the tip on page 51 for how to wash pesticides off produce.*

FARMED FISH

EXAMPLES	REASON TO AVOID
• Farmed salmon, shrimp, tilapia, carp, catfish	• According to a 2004 study in *Science*, farmed salmon is frequently contaminated with persistent organic pollutants such as PCBs and dioxin, which are harmful to our health

Foods to Avoid

INDUSTRIAL SEED OILS

EXAMPLES	REASON TO AVOID
• Include canola, corn, cottonseed, safflower, soybean, and peanut oils • Found in many processed foods and restaurant foods	• Highly inflammatory, processed, and potentially contaminated with industrial solvents

MILK

EXAMPLES	REASON TO AVOID
• Skim, 1%, 2%, and whole milk • Found in many processed foods	• Potentially inflammatory and difficult for many people to digest

PROCESSED FOODS

EXAMPLES	REASON TO AVOID
• Chicken nuggets, pizza, chips, margarine, fast food	• Low in nutrients and high in carbohydrates and oxidized fats, which trigger inflammation

REFINED CARBOHYDRATES

EXAMPLES	REASON TO AVOID
• Found in many processed foods, including baked goods (cakes, muffins, croissants), candy, and fruit juice • Sugars: white and brown sugars, sucrose, barley malt, high-fructose corn syrup, maltose, rice syrup, etc.	• Promote the growth of inflammatory gut bacteria and systemic inflammation • Suppress the immune system

SUGAR-SWEETENED BEVERAGES	
EXAMPLES	**REASON TO AVOID**
• Soda, juice, sports drinks, energy drinks	• Promote an inflammatory gut microbiota • Cause dramatic blood sugar swings • Impair brain function

TAP WATER	
EXAMPLES	**REASON TO AVOID**
• Water straight from the faucet • Bottled water (which is often just tap water that has been relabeled)	• Frequently contains environmental toxins such as heavy metals, pesticide residues, pharmaceutical drug residues, and plastic breakdown products

How to wash pesticides off produce

I've searched high and low for proven ways to wash pesticides and herbicides off produce. I recently found a science-based, quick, and effective strategy for accomplishing this goal—a baking soda bath!

To wash pesticides off your produce, first fill a large bowl with filtered water and 1 teaspoon of aluminum-free baking soda. Add your fruits and/or vegetables to the bath and let them soak for 10 to 15 minutes. After 10 to 15 minutes are up, pour off the water and rinse the produce under filtered water to remove any remaining baking soda.

Preparing for Success

Essential kitchen equipment

Here are the tools you'll need to set yourself up for success with the Detox Diet:

VEGETABLE PEELER, WOODEN CUTTING BOARD, CHEF'S KNIFE

Since you'll be eating lots of vegetables on the diet, consider investing in a vegetable peeler, a nice wooden cutting board, and a chef's knife for chopping veggies. Keep in mind that, according to the *Journal of Food Protection*, plastic cutting boards are frequently treated with triclosan, a synthetic antibacterial agent linked to gut microbiome disruption, and may harbor more bacteria than wooden cutting boards.

MEASURING CUPS, MEASURING SPOONS, AND MIXING BOWLS

These items will come in handy for measuring spices and baking healthy treats at home.

SLOTTED SPOONS, WOODEN SPOONS, SPATULA, AND LADLE

Whether you're making scrambled eggs for breakfast or a comforting stew for dinner, these items will be used repeatedly in your kitchen. I recommend using wooden spoons instead of metal or plastic because plastic utensils may degrade over time, releasing plasticizers into your food, and metal utensils can damage the surface of your pots and pans.

COOKWARE AND BAKEWARE

- Sauté pan
- Skillet
- Glass or ceramic baking dishes (avoid nonstick pans)
- Stockpot
- Soup pot

SLOW COOKER

If you don't already have a slow cooker, go out and buy one—it will quickly become your best friend! Slow cookers are great for making delicious, healthy meals with minimum amounts of effort and time. Simply add vegetables, a cut of meat, spices, and some filtered water to your slow cooker in the morning, and you can have a wonderful meal waiting for you when you get home at the end of the day.

I recommend storing food in glass rather than plastic containers because plastic containers frequently contain BPA and phthalates. BPA and phthalates are known to harm beneficial gut microbes, alter hormones, and adversely affect the brain.

- Food processor
- Blender
- Immersion blender (great for making soup)
- Mason jars (for bringing smoothies and salads to work)
- Dehydrator
- Juicer
- Mortar and pestle (for grinding herbs)

Pantry essentials

Keeping a well-stocked pantry will ensure that you always have healthy ingredients on hand to make a satisfying meal or snack.

Here are the items you should keep stocked at all times:

Coconut oil: Coconut oil is great for baking and other forms of cooking that involve high heat, such as roasting.

Olive oil: Olive oil combined with balsamic vinegar makes for a quick, healthy salad dressing. You can also use it in pasta sauces and for light sautéing.

Healthy flours: If you do a lot of baking, keep some healthy flours, such as almond flour, coconut flour, tapioca starch, and oat flour, on hand.

Gluten-free whole grains and beans: Oats, brown rice, wild rice, quinoa, buckwheat, chickpeas, lentils

Canned coconut milk: Canned coconut milk is a common ingredient in dairy-free baked goods, smoothies, and creamy sauces, so I recommend always keeping some on hand.

Balsamic vinegar and/or apple cider vinegar: These vinegars are great for making quick salad dressings or marinades for meat.

Spices and seasonings: Black peppercorns, cinnamon, garlic, oregano, thyme, cumin, turmeric, etc.

Nuts, nut butter, and seeds: Almonds, walnuts, macadamia nuts, cashews, hazelnuts, chia seeds, whole flaxseed (keep them refrigerated and grind in a coffee grinder immediately before using), hemp seeds, coconut flakes

Dried fruit: Raisins, cranberries, dates, figs, apples

Natural sweeteners: Coconut sugar, date sugar, raw honey, pure maple syrup, stevia, monk fruit (*luo han guo*) extract

Odds and ends: Baking soda (aluminum-free), baking powder, cream of tartar, xanthan gum or guar gum

Ten handy perishables

Keep the following items stocked in your fridge or freezer at all times:

1. **Cruciferous vegetables:** These vegetables are nutrient powerhouses and hold up well to food prep and reheating. Buy bulk bags of frozen cauliflower, broccoli, and Brussels sprouts at Costco or another big box store to save money.

2. **Leafy greens:** Keep a variety of leafy greens, such as romaine lettuce and chard, on hand for making salads and adding to sandwiches and wraps. Leafy greens will keep in your fridge for up to a week and should be stored in the crisper drawer to keep them fresh.

3. **Fresh fruit:** Fresh fruit makes for a portable, healthy snack as well as a great topping for salads, pancakes, and oatmeal. Buy fresh or frozen and try to pick in-season fruit.

4. **Eggs:** Eggs are an affordable, nutrient-dense protein source. If possible, look for eggs from hens that are allowed to graze on pasture, as these will contain a much higher omega-3 fatty acid content than eggs from corn- and soy-fed hens.

5. **Organic/grass-fed meats:** Meat is a satiating, nutrient-dense food that can quickly be made into a delicious meal on the stovetop or in a slow cooker.

6. **Organic poultry:** Buy a bulk package of organic chicken breasts to keep on hand for slow cooking or baking in the oven.

7. **Wild-caught seafood:** Keep some frozen wild salmon or mackerel fillets in your freezer. Buying these in bulk is a lot more affordable than buying fresh wild-caught fish.

8. **Starchy vegetables:** Keep sweet potatoes, winter squash, beets, and other starchy vegetables on hand. Roast or bake them for an easy side for dinner.

9. **Fresh herbs:** Growing your own fresh herbs is an affordable way to add zest to any meal.

10. **Dairy-free milks:** Keep almond, cashew, or coconut milk on hand for making smoothies or drinking plain.

Effort-saving tips

The best way to save time and effort in the kitchen is to meal prep! Meal prepping refers to the process of preparing whole meals or dishes ahead of schedule. Having prepared meals on hand will reduce the stress of having to cook throughout the week. It will also reduce the likelihood of you resorting to processed foods and fast food in a pinch!

There's no hard and fast rule for when and how often you should meal prep. Depending on your schedule, family size, and lifestyle, you can either prep meals a week at a time, a few days at a time, or a day in advance. Whichever strategy you choose, you'll increase your odds of sticking to a healthy eating pattern.

Need meal-prepping guidance? Check out the following apps that are specifically designed to assist you with meal prepping:

REAL PLANS

- Real Plans creates and organizes recipes and generates a weekly menu, grocery lists, and a day-by-day road map for getting healthy, delicious food on the table.

- A subscription will give you access to all meal plans (classic healthy, dairy-free, gluten-free, Paleo, keto, AIP, and more) and over 1,500 recipes.

EMEALS

- eMeals finds and selects recipes for you, making it easy to get simple, healthy dinners on the table every night.

- Meal plans include recipes (main and side dishes), shopping lists, and step-by-step instructions.

- Shop yourself or choose to skip the grocery store by sending your shopping list to AmazonFresh, Walmart Grocery, Kroger ClickList, Shipt, or Instacart.

YUMMLY RECIPES AND RECIPE BOX

- Yummly allows you to browse beautifully photographed and easy-to-follow recipes and save them to your own digital cookbook.

- Yummly's proprietary Food Genome and patent-pending Food Intelligence technology allow them to understand recipes at a deeper level and recommend recipes to users based on their diets, allergies, tastes, and more.

ADDITIONAL TIME-SAVING TIPS

- Print out your favorite healthy recipes from blogs and other websites and save them in a binder.

- Find 15 to 20 different recipes you enjoy and rotate them throughout the weeks.

- Make uncomplicated meals! You don't need to create a gourmet masterpiece at every meal. Keep things simple by combining high-quality protein, nonstarchy vegetables, and some healthy fat at each meal.

- Label and date leftovers so that you remember to use them up before they expire.

Traditional 30-Day Meal Plan

DAY 1

BREAKFAST:
Egg and Veggie Breakfast "Muffins" (page 68)

LUNCH:
Turmeric Chickpea Cauliflower Rice (page 92)

DINNER:
Beef and Veggie Stir-Fry (page 100)

DAY 2

BREAKFAST:
Noatmeal (page 71)

LUNCH:
Sesame Chicken Salad (page 80)

DINNER:
Kale, Lamb, and Sweet Potato Soup (page 115)

DAY 3

BREAKFAST:
Quinoa Breakfast Bars (page 72)

LUNCH:
Leftover Turmeric Chickpea Cauliflower Rice

DINNER:
Leftover Kale, Lamb, and Sweet Potato Soup

DAY 4

BREAKFAST:
Brain-Boosting Blueberry Smoothie (page 119)

LUNCH:
Leftover Sesame Chicken Salad

DINNER:
Leftover Beef and Veggie Stir-Fry

DAY 5

BREAKFAST:
Noatmeal

LUNCH:
Berry Chicken Mason Jar Salad (page 83)

DINNER:
Lemon-Garlic Salmon (page 112)

DAY 6

BREAKFAST:
Egg and Veggie Breakfast "Muffins"

LUNCH:
Leftover Lemon-Garlic Salmon

DINNER:
Burgers and Sweet Potato Fries (page 106)

DAY 7

BREAKFAST:
Whole-Grain Flax Waffles with Strawberry Purée (page 76)

LUNCH:
Leftover Berry Chicken Mason Jar Salad

DINNER:
Stuffed Bell Peppers (page 114)

DAY 8

BREAKFAST:
Breakfast Hash (page 70)

LUNCH:
Turkey Club Wrap (page 84)

DINNER:
Slow Cooker Chicken Tacos (page 109)

DAY 9

BREAKFAST:
Leftover Breakfast Hash

LUNCH:
Leftover Slow Cooker Chicken Tacos

DINNER:
Grain-Free Shepherd's Pie (page 101)

Traditional 30-Day Meal Plan

DAY 10	DAY 11	DAY 12
BREAKFAST: Green Smoothie (page 120)	**BREAKFAST:** Green Smoothie	**BREAKFAST:** Strawberry Overnight Oats (page 73)
LUNCH: Leftover Grain-Free Shepherd's Pie	**LUNCH:** Chicken and Wild Rice Soup (page 85)	**LUNCH:** BLT Egg Lettuce Wraps (page 89)
DINNER: Spaghetti Squash "Pasta" with Meatballs and Marinara Sauce (page 103)	**DINNER:** Leftover Spaghetti Squash "Pasta" with Meatballs and Marinara Sauce	**DINNER:** Leftover Chicken and Wild Rice Soup + salad

DAY 13	DAY 14	DAY 15
BREAKFAST: Leftover Strawberry Overnight Oats	**BREAKFAST:** Brain-Boosting Blueberry Smoothie	**BREAKFAST:** Mushroom and Greens Quiche with Almond Flour Crust (page 74)
LUNCH: Curried Egg Salad (page 90)	**LUNCH:** Leftover Curried Egg Salad	**LUNCH:** Cashew Tuna Salad (page 94)
DINNER: Beef and Veggie Stir-Fry	**DINNER:** Leftover Beef and Veggie Stir-Fry	**DINNER:** Red Lentil Dal (page 110)

DAY 16	DAY 17	DAY 18
BREAKFAST: Leftover Mushroom and Greens Quiche with Almond Flour Crust	**BREAKFAST:** Quinoa Breakfast Bars	**BREAKFAST:** Green Smoothie
LUNCH: Cold Asian Zucchini Noodles with Chicken (page 88)	**LUNCH:** Leftover Cold Asian Zucchini Noodles with Chicken	**LUNCH:** Taco Salad (page 82)
DINNER: Slow Cooker Sloppy Joes (page 108)	**DINNER:** Leftover Red Lentil Dal	**DINNER:** Balsamic Chicken with Brussels Sprouts and Bacon (page 105)

Traditional 30-Day Meal Plan

DAY 19

BREAKFAST:
Quinoa Breakfast Bars

LUNCH:
Leftover Balsamic Chicken with Brussels Sprouts and Bacon

DINNER:
Leftover Taco Salad + rice

DAY 20

BREAKFAST:
Green Smoothie

LUNCH:
BLT Egg Lettuce Wraps Plantain Chips (page 122)

DINNER:
Simple Fish Curry (page 113)

DAY 21

BREAKFAST:
Strawberry Overnight Oats

LUNCH:
Leftover Simple Fish Curry

DINNER:
Stuffed Bell Peppers

DAY 22

BREAKFAST:
Egg and Veggie Breakfast "Muffins"

LUNCH:
Hearty Vegetable Soup (page 86)

DINNER:
Zucchini Noodles with Peas

DAY 23

BREAKFAST:
Egg and Veggie Breakfast "Muffins"

LUNCH:
Leftover Stuffed Bell Peppers

DINNER:
Chinese Chicken Salad with Cauliflower Rice (page 98)

DAY 24

BREAKFAST:
Breakfast Hash

LUNCH:
Leftover Chinese Chicken Salad with Cauliflower Rice

DINNER:
Kale, Lamb, and Sweet Potato Soup

DAY 25

BREAKFAST:
Leftover Breakfast Hash

LUNCH:
Balsamic Roasted Root Veggie Salad (page 81)

DINNER:
Leftover Kale, Lamb, and Sweet Potato Soup

DAY 26

BREAKFAST:
Brain-Boosting Blueberry Smoothie

LUNCH:
Butternut Squash Chili (page 87)

DINNER:
Lemon-Garlic Salmon

DAY 27

BREAKFAST:
Noatmeal

LUNCH:
Berry Chicken Mason Jar Salad

DINNER:
Leftover Lemon-Garlic Salmon

Traditional 30-Day Meal Plan

DAY 28	DAY 29	DAY 30
BREAKFAST: Whole-Grain Flax Waffles with Strawberry Purée	**BREAKFAST:** Green Smoothie	**BREAKFAST:** Noatmeal
LUNCH: Sweet Potato Ramen Bowl (page 95)	**LUNCH:** Turmeric Chickpea Cauliflower Rice	**LUNCH:** BLT Egg Lettuce Wraps
DINNER: Grain-Free Shepherd's Pie	**DINNER:** Leftover Sweet Potato Ramen Bowl	**DINNER:** Leftover Turmeric Chickpea Cauliflower Rice

Vegetarian & Vegan 30-Day Meal Plan

DAY 1	DAY 2	DAY 3
BREAKFAST: Egg and Veggie Breakfast "Muffins" (omit bacon/sausage) (page 68)	**BREAKFAST:** Leftover Egg and Veggie Breakfast "Muffins"	**BREAKFAST:** Noatmeal Ⓥ (page 71)
LUNCH: Hearty Vegetable Soup Ⓥ (page 86)	**LUNCH:** Leftover Club Wrap Ⓥ	**LUNCH:** BLT Egg Lettuce Wraps (omit bacon) (page 89)
DINNER: Club Wrap Ⓥ (sub tempeh or tofu for the turkey) (page 84)	**DINNER:** Red Lentil Dal Ⓥ (page 110)	**DINNER:** Stuffed Bell Peppers Ⓥ (page 114)

DAY 4	DAY 5	DAY 6
BREAKFAST: Quinoa Breakfast Bars Ⓥ (page 72)	**BREAKFAST:** Brain-Boosting Blueberry Smoothie Ⓥ (page 119)	**BREAKFAST:** Quinoa Breakfast Bars Ⓥ
LUNCH: Leftover Stuffed Bell Peppers Ⓥ	**LUNCH:** Sweet Potato Ramen Bowl (page 95)	**LUNCH:** Leftover Slow Cooker Tacos Ⓥ
DINNER: Slow Cooker Tacos Ⓥ (sub beans for the chicken) (page 109)	**DINNER:** Leftover Slow Cooker Tacos Ⓥ (omit chicken)	**DINNER:** Leftover Sweet Potato Ramen Bowl

Vegetarian & Vegan 30-Day Meal Plan

DAY 7

BREAKFAST:
Green Smoothie Ⓥ (page 120)

LUNCH:
Turmeric Chickpea
Cauliflower Rice Ⓥ (page 92)

DINNER:
Leftover Red Lentil Dal Ⓥ

DAY 8

BREAKFAST:
Mushroom and Greens
Quiche with Almond Flour
Crust (page 74)

LUNCH:
Curried Egg Salad (page 90)

DINNER:
Stuffed Bell Peppers Ⓥ

DAY 9

BREAKFAST:
Leftover Mushroom and
Greens Quiche with Almond
Flour Crust

LUNCH:
Zucchini Noodles with Peas Ⓥ
(page 107)

DINNER:
Spaghetti Squash "Pasta" Ⓥ
(sub roasted vegetables for
the meatballs) (page 103)

DAY 10

BREAKFAST:
Strawberry Overnight Oats Ⓥ
(page 73)

LUNCH:
Cashew Salad (sub tofu
for tuna) (page 94)

DINNER:
Veggie Stir-Fry Ⓥ (sub
tempeh/tofu for the beef)
(page 100)

DAY 11

BREAKFAST:
Leftover Strawberry
Overnight Oats Ⓥ

LUNCH:
Leftover Veggie Stir-Fry Ⓥ

DINNER:
Hearty Vegetable Soup Ⓥ
(page 86)

DAY 12

BREAKFAST:
Green Smoothie Ⓥ

LUNCH:
Balsamic Roasted Root
Veggie Salad Ⓥ (page 81)
Plantain Chips Ⓥ (page 122)
Beet Hummus Ⓥ (page 123)

DINNER:
Stuffed Bell Peppers Ⓥ

DAY 13

BREAKFAST:
No-Bake Banana Chocolate
Chip Granola Bars Ⓥ
(page 118) with coconut or
almond milk yogurt

LUNCH:
Leftover Stuffed Bell
Peppers Ⓥ

DINNER:
Slow Cooker Sloppy Joes Ⓥ
(with vegan modification)
(page 108)

DAY 14

BREAKFAST:
Brain-Boosting Blueberry
Smoothie Ⓥ

LUNCH:
Grain-Free Shepherd's Pie
(sub brown or green lentils for
the meat) (page 101)

DINNER:
Leftover Slow Cooker Sloppy
Joes Ⓥ (with vegan
modification)

DAY 15

BREAKFAST:
Egg and Veggie Breakfast
"Muffins" (omit bacon/
sausage)

LUNCH:
Berry Mason Jar Salad Ⓥ
(sub chickpeas for the
chicken) (page 83)

DINNER:
Red Lentil Dal Ⓥ

Vegetarian & Vegan 30-Day Meal Plan

DAY 16

BREAKFAST:
Green Smoothie Ⓥ

LUNCH:
Leftover Red Lentil Dal Ⓥ

DINNER:
Taco Salad (omit beef)
(page 82)

DAY 17

BREAKFAST:
Egg and Veggie Breakfast
"Muffins" (omit bacon/
sausage)

LUNCH:
Leftover Taco Salad

DINNER:
Butternut Squash Chili Ⓥ
(sub beans for the meat and
vegetable broth for the beef
or chicken broth) (page 87)

DAY 18

BREAKFAST:
Noatmeal Ⓥ

LUNCH:
Cashew Salad (sub tofu for
the tuna) (page 94)

DINNER:
Sweet Potato Ramen Bowl

DAY 19

BREAKFAST:
Quinoa Breakfast Bars Ⓥ

LUNCH:
Leftover Sweet Potato
Ramen Bowl

DINNER:
Leftover Cashew Salad + rice

DAY 20

BREAKFAST:
Quinoa Breakfast Bars Ⓥ

LUNCH:
Cold Asian Zucchini Noodles
(sub tempeh or tofu for the
chicken) (page 88)

DINNER:
Stuffed Bell Peppers Ⓥ

DAY 21

BREAKFAST:
Brain-Boosting Blueberry
Smoothie Ⓥ

LUNCH:
Leftover Stuffed Bell
Peppers Ⓥ

DINNER:
Leftover Cold Asian Zucchini
Noodles

DAY 22

BREAKFAST:
Whole-Grain Flax Waffles
with Strawberry Purée
(page 76)

LUNCH:
BLT Egg Lettuce Wraps
(omit bacon)

DINNER:
Turmeric Chickpea
Cauliflower Rice Ⓥ

DAY 23

BREAKFAST:
Whole-Grain Flax Waffles
with Strawberry Purée

LUNCH:
Club Wrap (page 84)

DINNER:
Hearty Vegetable Soup Ⓥ
(page 86) + baked sweet
potato

DAY 24

BREAKFAST:
Mushroom and Greens
Quiche with Almond Flour
Crust

LUNCH:
Balsamic Roasted Root
Veggie Salad Ⓥ

DINNER:
Leftover Hearty Vegetable
Soup Ⓥ + baked sweet
potato

DAY 25	DAY 26	DAY 27
BREAKFAST: No-Bake Banana Chocolate Chip Granola Bars Ⓥ with coconut or almond milk yogurt	**BREAKFAST:** Noatmeal Ⓥ	**BREAKFAST:** Egg and Veggie Breakfast "Muffins" (omit bacon/sausage)
LUNCH: Leftover Balsamic Roasted Root Veggie Salad Ⓥ	**LUNCH:** Taco Salad (omit beef) (page 82)	**LUNCH:** Berry Mason Jar Salad Ⓥ (sub tofu/tempeh for the chicken)
DINNER: Leftover Hearty Vegetable Soup Ⓥ	**DINNER:** Sweet Potato Ramen Bowl	**DINNER:** Veggie Stir-Fry Ⓥ (sub tempeh/tofu for the beef)
DAY 28	**DAY 29**	**DAY 30**
BREAKFAST: Green Smoothie Ⓥ	**BREAKFAST:** Mushroom and Greens Quiche with Almond Flour Crust	**BREAKFAST:** Leftover Mushroom and Greens Quiche with Almond Flour Crust
LUNCH: Curried Egg Salad (page 90)	**LUNCH:** Cold Asian Zucchini Noodles (sub tempeh or tofu for the chicken)	**LUNCH:** Butternut Squash Chili Ⓥ (sub beans for the meat and vegetable broth for the beef or chicken broth)
DINNER: Slow Cooker Sloppy Joes Ⓥ (with vegan modification)	**DINNER:** Slow Cooker Tacos Ⓥ	**DINNER:** Leftover Slow Cooker Tacos Ⓥ

Ⓥ = Vegan

PART 3

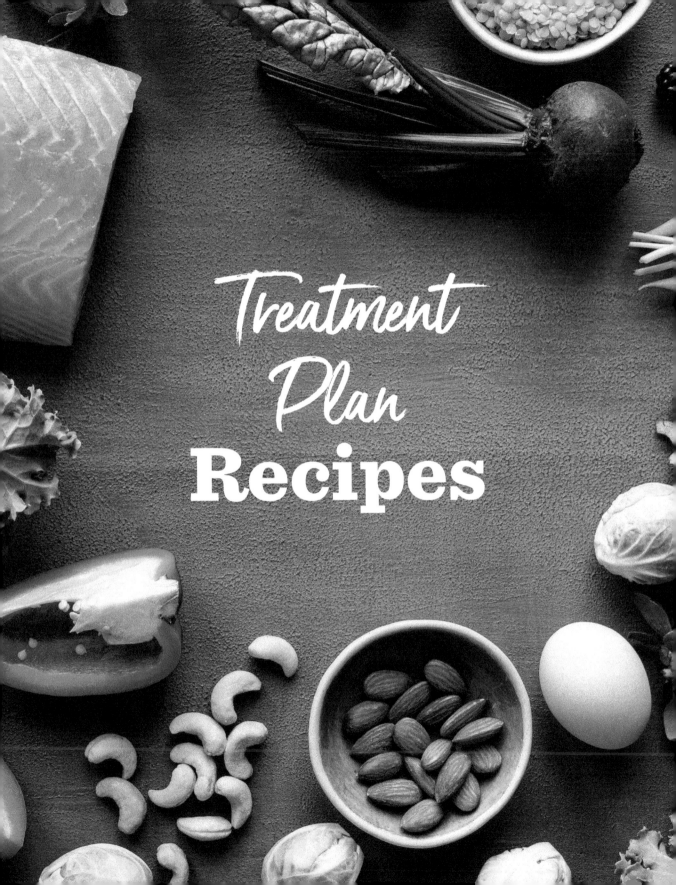

Treatment
Plan
Recipes

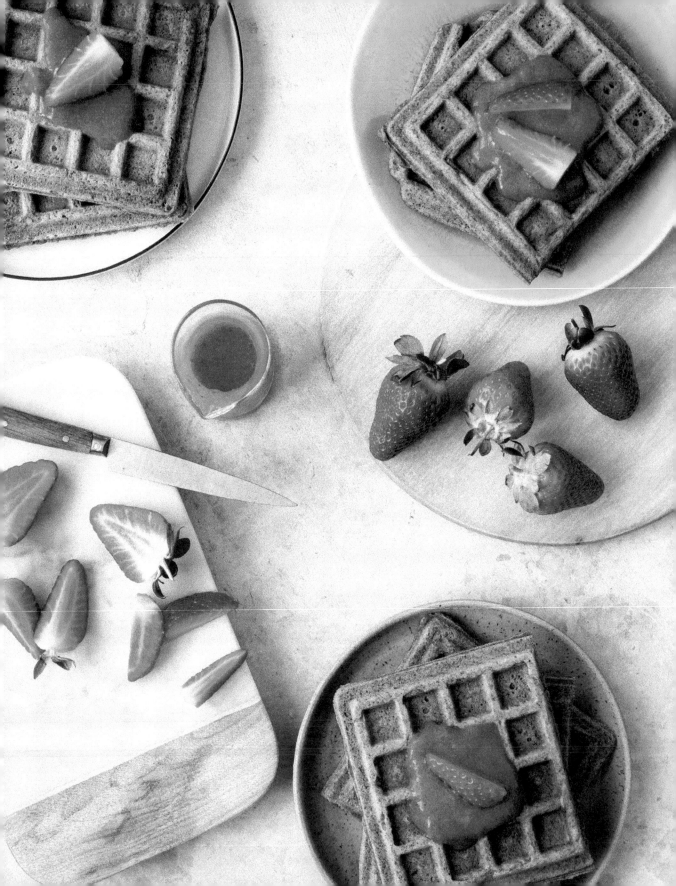

Chapter 4

Quick and Easy Breakfasts

When you're low on energy and wake up with brain fog, the last thing you want to do is spend any amount of time making a healthy breakfast. Enter: make-ahead recipes! Everything in this chapter can be prepped and/or cooked ahead of time and stored in your fridge or on the counter to make sure you start your days off right.

Egg *and* Veggie Breakfast "Muffins"

DAIRY-FREE, GLUTEN-FREE, UNDER 30 MINUTES

Are you always in a rush on weekday mornings? Do you find yourself reaching for sugary baked goods to complement your morning coffee because you didn't have time to make a wholesome breakfast? These healthy egg "muffins" are the perfect make-ahead, grab-and-go breakfast for anyone with a busy schedule. They are an excellent source of protein and healthy fats and will leave you feeling satiated and energetic all morning, without the sugar crash from eating sweet pastries for breakfast! **SERVES 4**

PREP TIME: 5 MINUTES
COOK TIME: 20 MINUTES

10 eggs

8 ounces pre-cooked bacon or sausage, chopped

1 bell pepper, diced

½ onion, finely diced

½ teaspoon fine sea salt

½ teaspoon freshly ground black pepper

2 tablespoons avocado oil or melted coconut oil

1. Preheat the oven to 375°F.

2. Crack the eggs into a large mixing bowl and whisk thoroughly. Add the chopped meat, bell pepper, onion, salt, and pepper, and mix.

3. Grease a stainless-steel muffin tin with the avocado oil. Alternately, you can use paper muffin liners.

4. Spoon the egg mixture into the muffin tin, evenly distributing it among all the cups. Put the full tin into the oven and bake for 20 minutes, or until the eggs are slightly golden brown on top and cooked all the way through.

5. Remove from the oven and allow to cool before eating. You can store the muffins in the fridge for up to 1 week or in the freezer if you don't plan to use all of them immediately.

Substitution Tip: To make this recipe vegetarian, omit the sausage/bacon.

How to make a flax "egg": A flax "egg" is a good substitute for real eggs in recipes that call for the binding properties of eggs. Here's how you can make a flax "egg" at home:

1. Mix 1 tablespoon of freshly ground flaxseed with 3 tablespoons of warm, filtered water in a small bowl. Stir thoroughly.

2. Place the bowl in the fridge for 15 minutes, until the flax "egg" has thickened.

3. Use the flax "egg" to replace real eggs in a 1:1 ratio (1 flax "egg" subs for 1 real egg).

Per Serving (2 muffins) Calories: 292; Total Fat: 20g; Saturated Fat: 10g; Sodium: 90mg; Carbohydrates: 6g; Fiber: 1g; Protein: 24g

Breakfast Hash

DAIRY-FREE, GLUTEN-FREE, VEGETARIAN OPTION

Looking for a savory, hearty, healthy breakfast? This delicious hash has you covered! A combination of sweet potatoes, nonstarchy veggies, eggs, sausage, and spices will thrill your taste buds and keep you full all morning long. **SERVES 4**

PREP TIME: 10 MINUTES
COOK TIME: 30 MINUTES

3 tablespoons avocado oil or coconut oil, divided

8 ounces sausage

1 medium onion, chopped

1 bell pepper, chopped

½ teaspoon smoked paprika

Fine sea salt

Freshly ground black pepper

2 sweet potatoes, chopped into ½-inch cubes

4 eggs

1. Preheat the oven to 400°F.

2. Heat a large cast-iron or enamel skillet over medium heat and pour in 1 tablespoon of avocado oil, coating the bottom of the pan. Once the oil is heated, add the sausage to the pan, crumbling it and stirring until evenly browned.

3. When the sausage is 75 percent done, add the onion and bell pepper. Cook with the sausage until the onion and pepper are soft and fragrant. Remove from the heat and set aside.

4. In a separate skillet, add the remaining 2 tablespoons of oil, the paprika, and a dash of salt and pepper. Add the chopped sweet potatoes, stir to coat with the oil, and cook until the potatoes are soft.

5. Transfer the softened potatoes to the skillet with the sausage, onion, and pepper. Spread out the meat and veggie mixture evenly and then make four small indents in the surface of the mixture. Crack an egg into each indent.

6. Place the skillet into the oven and bake for 10 to 15 minutes, until the eggs are thoroughly cooked.

7. Remove the skillet from the oven and allow to cool for 5 to 10 minutes before serving. The hash will keep in an airtight container in the refrigerator for up to 1 week.

Substitution Tip: To make this recipe vegetarian, omit the sausage.

Per Serving (1 bowl of hash with 1 egg)
Calories: 398; Total Fat: 30g; Saturated Fat: 15g; Sodium: 514mg; Carbohydrates: 18g; Fiber: 3g; Protein: 16g

Noatmeal

DAIRY-FREE, GLUTEN-FREE, UNDER 30 MINUTES, VEGETARIAN, VEGAN

Noatmeal (oatmeal with no oats!) is a nutrient-dense play on the classic breakfast staple. This dish is equally delicious hot or cold in the morning and is rich in fiber and micronutrients. SERVES 1

PREP TIME: 5 MINUTES
COOK TIME: 1 TO 2 MINUTES

½ ripe banana

2 tablespoons shredded coconut

2 tablespoons almond flour, coconut flour, or tigernut flour

½ cup unsweetened almond or coconut milk

¼ teaspoon ground cinnamon

1 tablespoon pure maple syrup

Pinch fine sea salt

Toppings of choice: berries, chopped almonds or walnuts

1. Mash the banana with a fork or potato masher in the bottom of a microwave-safe bowl. Add the coconut, flour, almond milk, cinnamon, maple syrup, and salt and stir to combine.

2. Microwave the noatmeal until hot and bubbling. Remove from the microwave, stir, and let stand for a couple minutes before eating. Alternately, you can heat the noatmeal on your stovetop in a saucepan.

3. Top your noatmeal with berries, chopped almonds or walnuts, or any other favorite toppings, and serve.

Substitution Tip: Replace the maple syrup with Lakanto monk fruit sweetener if you want a lower-carb version.

Per Serving (1 small bowl) Calories: 183; Total Fat: 7g; Saturated Fat: 3g; Sodium: 330mg; Carbohydrates: 31g; Fiber: 4g; Protein: 2g

Quinoa Breakfast Bars

DAIRY-FREE, GLUTEN-FREE, VEGETARIAN, VEGAN OPTION

Breakfast bars are a convenient, nutrient-dense, on-the-go breakfast for busy individuals. They also make a delicious snack! **MAKES 12 BARS**

PREP TIME: 15 MINUTES
COOK TIME: 40 MINUTES

Avocado oil or melted coconut oil, for greasing

1½ cups old-fashioned rolled oats (choose gluten-free oats such as Bob's Red Mill if you are gluten-sensitive)

1½ cups cooked quinoa

1 tablespoon ground cinnamon

1 teaspoon baking powder

½ teaspoon baking soda

¼ teaspoon fine sea salt

1 cup unsweetened almond or coconut milk

¼ cup pure maple syrup or honey

3 tablespoons almond butter or cashew butter

1 large egg

1 teaspoon vanilla extract

1¼ cups blueberries, raspberries, or chopped strawberries

1. Preheat the oven to 350°F with a rack in the center position.

2. Lightly coat an 8-by-8-inch square stainless-steel baking pan or glass baking dish with oil. You can also line the pan with parchment paper, ensuring that it extends beyond the pan's edges.

3. In a medium bowl, combine the oats, quinoa, cinnamon, baking powder, baking soda, and salt. In a separate bowl, mix together the almond milk, maple syrup, nut butter, egg, and vanilla.

4. Slowly pour the wet ingredients into the dry mixture and stir with a silicone spatula or spoon to combine. Gently fold the berries into the mixture.

5. Pour the mixture into the prepared baking pan and bake for 35 to 40 minutes, until the bars are golden brown and a toothpick inserted into the bars comes out clean.

6. Remove the pan from the oven. If you used the parchment option, lift the edges of the paper and transfer the baked mixture to a wire cooling rack. Let the mixture cool completely before cutting into bars.

Substitution Tip: Substitute a flax "egg" (see page 69) for the real egg to make the recipe vegan.

Per Serving (1 bar) Calories: 109; Total Fat: 4g; Saturated Fat: 1g; Sodium: 99mg; Carbohydrates: 16g; Fiber: 2g; Protein: 3g

Strawberry Overnight Oats

DAIRY-FREE, GLUTEN-FREE, VEGETARIAN, VEGAN

Overnight oats are the perfect make-ahead breakfast! All the prep occurs the night before, and the prep itself is minimal. There are countless ways to customize your overnight oats using fresh or frozen fruits, chopped nuts and seeds, and nut butter. **SERVES 1**

PREP TIME: 5 MINUTES

½ cup rolled oats (gluten-free if necessary)

½ cup almond or coconut milk

¼ cup sliced strawberries

½ teaspoon vanilla extract

½ teaspoon ground cinnamon

½ teaspoon pure maple syrup or honey

1. Combine all the ingredients in an 8-ounce Mason jar with a lid. Stir the mixture well.

2. Place the Mason jar in the fridge for at least 4 to 5 hours, but preferably overnight. This will allow the oats to soak up the milk and flavors of the vanilla, cinnamon, and maple syrup.

3. You can reheat the overnight oats in the morning, if you want, either in a saucepan on the stovetop or in the microwave.

Per Serving Calories: 213; Total Fat: 4g; Saturated Fat: 0g; Sodium: 78mg; Carbohydrates: 37g; Fiber: 6g; Protein: 7g

Mushroom *and* Greens Quiche *with* Almond Flour Crust

DAIRY-FREE, GLUTEN-FREE, VEGETARIAN

Quiche may seem like a fancy, complicated breakfast recipe, but this version transforms the classic dish into a simple, healthy meal that requires only a small amount of prep time. I recommend making this quiche on Sunday night so you can eat it all throughout the week. **SERVES 6**

PREP TIME: 20 MINUTES
COOK TIME: 50 MINUTES

FOR THE CRUST

⅓ cup avocado oil or olive oil, plus more
   for greasing

2 cups almond flour

3 garlic cloves, minced

1 tablespoon minced fresh thyme

½ teaspoon fine sea salt

¼ teaspoon freshly ground black pepper

1 tablespoon plus 1 teaspoon filtered water

FOR THE FILLING

Avocado oil, for greasing

1½ cups sliced mushrooms

½ medium onion, chopped

½ teaspoon fine sea salt, plus a pinch

3 cups chopped greens, such as arugula
   or spinach

6 large eggs

⅓ cup unsweetened almond milk

TO MAKE THE CRUST

1. Preheat the oven to 400°F. Grease a cast-iron or enamel skillet or 9-inch pie pan with avocado oil.

2. In a large mixing bowl, stir together the almond flour, garlic, thyme, salt, and pepper. Add the oil and water and mix until thoroughly combined. Alternatively, mix the dough in a food processor.

3. Roll the dough roughly into a ball shape and transfer to the greased skillet or pie pan. Press the dough until it is evenly spread across the bottom and at least 1 inch up the sides. Bake the dough until it has a light golden-brown crust, about 20 minutes.

TO MAKE THE FILLING

1. In a separate skillet over medium heat, heat enough avocado oil to coat the pan. Add the mushrooms, onion, and a pinch of salt, cooking until they are soft. Add the greens, cooking until wilted (30 seconds to a minute at most).

2. In another large mixing bowl, whisk the eggs, almond milk, and remaining ½ teaspoon of salt. Stir in the mushroom and greens mixture.

3. Pour the egg and veggie mixture into the baked almond flour crust. Bake for 30 minutes, or until a toothpick inserted into the quiche comes out clean. If you plan to eat some quiche immediately, let it cool for 20 minutes before slicing. Store leftovers in an airtight container in the refrigerator for up to 4 days.

Per Serving (1 slice) Calories: 312; Total Fat: 27g; Saturated Fat: 4g; Sodium: 156mg; Carbohydrates: 8g; Fiber: 3g; Protein: 12g

Whole-Grain Flax Waffles *with* Strawberry Purée

VEGETARIAN, UNDER 30 MINUTES

Waffles are a breakfast tradition. They are also frequently full of refined carbohydrates and added sugars, which, unfortunately, do not support optimal health. This recipe offers a healthier take on waffles, using whole-wheat pastry flour and flaxseed instead of white pastry flour. The end results are waffles that are crisp on the outside and fluffy and tender on the inside. The strawberry purée is a more nutritious, lower-sugar alternative to syrup and provides a tangy sweetness that goes perfectly with the waffles!

SERVES 6

PREP TIME: 15 MINUTES
COOK TIME: 15 MINUTES

FOR THE PURÉE

1 quart strawberries, hulled and chopped

1 cup water

2 tablespoons honey

½ teaspoon vanilla extract

FOR THE WAFFLES

2¼ cups whole-wheat pastry flour

¼ cup ground flaxseed

2½ teaspoons baking powder

1 teaspoon baking soda

½ teaspoon kosher or sea salt

2 teaspoons ground cinnamon

2 tablespoons dark brown sugar

¼ cup avocado oil or melted coconut oil

3 large eggs

2 teaspoons vanilla extract

1 cup unsweetened almond milk or coconut milk

Avocado oil or coconut oil cooking spray, for preparing the waffle iron

TO MAKE THE PURÉE

Place the strawberries, water, honey, and vanilla in a medium saucepan. Bring to a simmer and cook for 5 to 6 minutes, until the strawberries are soft. Use an immersion blender to purée the strawberries or transfer the mixture to a blender and purée until smooth.

TO MAKE THE WAFFLES

1.   In a medium mixing bowl, whisk together the flour, flaxseed, baking powder, baking soda, and salt until combined.

2.   In a large mixing bowl, whisk together the cinnamon, brown sugar, and avocado oil until well combined. Whisk in one egg at a time until the mixture is fluffy. Add the vanilla and milk and whisk until combined. Slowly whisk the dry ingredients into the wet mixture.

3.   Heat a Belgian waffle maker over medium heat. Once hot, coat with cooking spray. Evenly spoon ⅔ cup of batter into the waffle maker. Shut the lid and cook for 1½ to 2 minutes until the waffle is browned on the outside. Repeat with the remaining batter.

4. Serve the waffles with strawberry purée. Store leftover waffles in the refrigerator in an airtight glass storage container or wrapped in parchment paper and sealed in a plastic bag for up to 5 days. Serve chilled or reheat in the microwave on high power for 30 seconds. Store the strawberry purée in an airtight glass container for up to 5 days.

Substitution Tips: Gluten-free all-purpose flour can be substituted for regular flour to make this recipe gluten-free. Try oat flour for a higher-fiber gluten-free version of these waffles. Use raspberries or blueberries instead of strawberries to make the fruit purée. You can make this recipe vegan by substituting flax "eggs" for the real eggs (see page 69).

Cooking Tip: To make waffle batter into pancake batter, reduce the oil to 2 tablespoons (instead of ¼ cup), and cook in a greased nonstick skillet over medium heat for 1 to 2 minutes per side until set.

Make It a Meal: This recipe can be served with lower-sodium chicken sausages or bacon for a higher-protein meal.

Per Serving (2 standard-size waffles) Calories: 457; Total Fat: 15g; Saturated Fat: 2g; Sodium: 437mg; Carbohydrates: 68g; Fiber: 11g; Protein: 14g

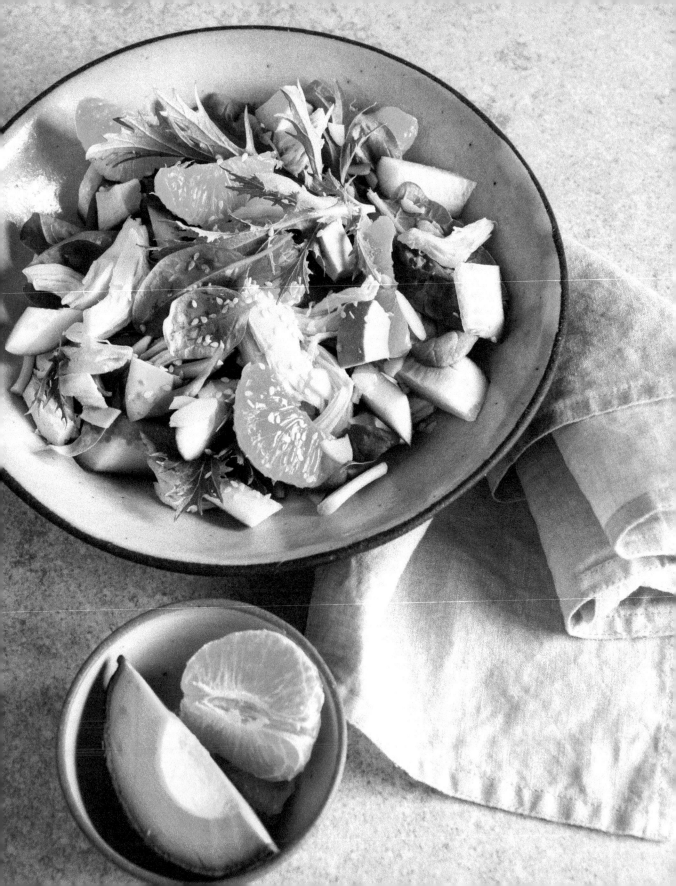

Chapter 5

Healthy Lunches

Your lunch can either help you soar through the rest of your day with abundant energy or send you into a blood sugar crash and afternoon slump, depending on what you choose to eat. In the healthy lunches featured in this chapter, I've included recipes rich in protein, healthy fats, and vegetables, with moderate amounts of carbs; these meals were strategically planned to help you sustain a good energy level throughout the afternoon, reducing your need for a sugary or caffeinated pick-me-up mid-afternoon. As a result, you'll see traditional sandwiches reimagined as veggie-based wraps, a variety of salads, and numerous protein options.

Sesame Chicken Salad

DAIRY-FREE, GLUTEN-FREE, UNDER 30 MINUTES

This refreshing salad manages to be both sweet and savory, with a lovely crunch thanks to the addition of slivered almonds. It requires very little prep time, especially if you make the shredded chicken ahead of time in a slow cooker. **SERVES 1**

PREP TIME: 10 MINUTES

FOR THE SALAD

3 cups mixed greens

4 ounces cooked chicken breast, shredded

2 tablespoons slivered almonds

½ cup sliced cucumber

1 cup fresh orange segments

2 scallions, chopped

FOR THE DRESSING

1 tablespoon toasted sesame seeds

1 teaspoon peeled and grated fresh ginger root

2 tablespoons tamari sauce

2 tablespoons rice vinegar

1 tablespoon honey

1 scallion, finely chopped

Juice of ½ lime

⅓ cup extra-virgin olive oil

¼ cup freshly squeezed orange juice

2 teaspoons toasted sesame oil

1. In a large mixing bowl, combine the greens, chicken, almonds, cucumber, orange, and scallions.

2. In a glass jar or other lidded container, combine the sesame seeds, ginger, tamari sauce, rice vinegar, honey, scallions, lime juice, olive oil, orange juice, and sesame oil. Cover and shake well.

3. Add the dressing to the salad and gently toss to coat.

4. Serve immediately or refrigerate the salad and dressing in separate airtight containers for up to 2 days.

Per Serving Calories: 364; Total Fat: 8g; Saturated Fat: 1g; Sodium: 654mg; Carbohydrates: 42g; Fiber: 10g; Protein: 35g

Balsamic Roasted Root Veggie Salad

DAIRY-FREE, GLUTEN-FREE, VEGETARIAN, VEGAN

This hearty salad has a surprising burst of flavors and textures. It tastes great warm or chilled and will no doubt become a lunch staple in your diet! **SERVES 4**

PREP TIME: 20 MINUTES
COOK TIME: 20 MINUTES

2 medium carrots, peeled and chopped into small chunks

1 medium zucchini, cubed

8 ounces mushrooms, sliced

1 small red onion, sliced

4 garlic cloves, minced

2 tablespoons olive oil

2 tablespoons balsamic vinegar

½ teaspoon dried rosemary

Fine sea salt

¼ teaspoon freshly ground black pepper

1½ cups cooked quinoa (made from about ½ cup dry quinoa)

Mixed greens, for serving

¼ cup sliced almonds or walnuts

1. Preheat the oven to 400°F.

2. Place the carrots, zucchini, mushrooms, onion, and garlic on a baking sheet and toss with the olive oil, vinegar, rosemary, salt, and pepper until evenly coated.

3. Bake for 20 minutes, or until the carrots are tender. Toss halfway through the baking time to make sure the vegetables bake evenly.

4. Place the quinoa in a large bowl and fluff it with a fork. Add the roasted vegetables and toss to combine.

5. Top the mixed greens with the roasted vegetable and quinoa mixture. Top with almonds or walnuts. Serve warm or chilled.

Per Serving (1 salad) Calories: 227; Total Fat: 12g; Saturated Fat: 1g; Sodium: 123mg; Carbohydrates: 26g; Fiber: 5g; Protein: 8g

Taco Salad

DAIRY-FREE, GLUTEN-FREE, UNDER 30 MINUTES

Taco salad is a delicious way to fit a bunch of veggies into your lunch alongside the wonderful flavors of Mexican cuisine! I like to eat my taco salad with homemade Plantain Chips (page 122). SERVES 4

PREP TIME: 10 MINUTES
COOK TIME: 10 MINUTES

FOR THE TACO MEAT

½ teaspoon garlic powder

½ teaspoon onion powder

½ teaspoon smoked or regular paprika

1 teaspoon dried oregano

1 teaspoon fine sea salt

1 teaspoon freshly ground black pepper

2 teaspoons ground cumin

1 tablespoon chili powder

1 pound ground beef

1 tablespoon avocado oil

FOR THE SALAD

1 head romaine lettuce, chopped

1 cup cherry tomatoes, halved

½ cup prepared salsa

1 cup prepared guacamole

TO MAKE THE TACO MEAT

1. In a medium bowl, combine the garlic powder, onion powder, paprika, oregano, salt, pepper, cumin, and chili powder with the ground beef. Mix thoroughly.

2. Heat a large skillet over medium heat, adding enough avocado oil to coat it evenly. Add the seasoned ground beef and cook for 10 minutes, breaking up the beef into small chunks. Cook until the moisture has evaporated from the pan.

TO MAKE THE SALAD

In a large bowl, combine the lettuce and tomatoes. Add the taco meat and top with salsa and guacamole.

Per Serving (1 salad) Calories: 305; Total Fat: 18g; Saturated Fat: 4g; Sodium: 772mg; Carbohydrates: 16g; Fiber: 6g; Protein: 26g

Berry Chicken Mason Jar Salad

DAIRY-FREE, GLUTEN-FREE, UNDER 30 MINUTES

Mason jar salads are a convenient, fun way to bring a salad to work for lunch. This salad makes use of one of my favorite foods, berries, which are anti-inflammatory powerhouses that support a healthy gut, immune system, and brain. Make a batch of chicken breasts ahead of time to use in this salad and in the other recipes within this chapter. When putting together the salad in the Mason jar, layer the ingredients to create an especially photogenic meal! **SERVES 1**

PREP TIME: 15 MINUTES

FOR THE DRESSING

1 cup mixed berries (blueberries, strawberries, raspberries, blackberries)

¼ cup balsamic vinegar

2 tablespoons freshly squeezed lemon juice

1 tablespoon pure maple syrup

⅓ cup olive oil

Fine sea salt

Freshly ground black pepper

FOR THE SALAD

2 to 3 tablespoons dressing (above)

1 cup cubed cooked chicken

½ cup arugula

½ cup mixed berries

¼ cup sliced almonds

TO MAKE THE DRESSING

Put the berries, vinegar, lemon juice, maple syrup, and olive oil in a blender or food processor and mix until smooth. Taste and then add the desired amount of salt and pepper.

TO MAKE THE SALAD

Pour 2 to 3 tablespoons of the dressing in the bottom of a Mason jar. Add the chicken, arugula, mixed berries, and almonds. Store in the refrigerator until lunchtime. Mix with a fork and enjoy!

Per Serving Calories: 560; Total Fat: 33g; Saturated Fat: 5g; Sodium: 119mg; Carbohydrates: 17g; Fiber: 6g; Protein: 49g

Turkey Club Wrap

DAIRY-FREE, UNDER 30 MINUTES

This turkey club wrap is a light but satiating spring and summer meal. You can either use tortillas for your wrap or, to make a lower-carb version, substitute collard greens for the tortillas. **SERVES 1**

PREP TIME: 5 MINUTES

1 tortilla wrap or 2 collard green leaves

1 tablespoon Avocado Oil Mayonnaise
   (page 91)

1 teaspoon mustard

2 ounces turkey cold cuts

2 cooked bacon slices

¼ avocado, sliced

2 slices beefsteak or Roma tomato

1 cup shredded romaine lettuce

1. Place the tortilla on a work surface. Spread it with mayonnaise and mustard and layer on the turkey, bacon, avocado, tomato, and lettuce.

2. Wrap the ingredients in the tortilla, cut, and serve.

Per Serving (1 large tortilla) Calories: 477; Total Fat: 29g; Saturated Fat: 7g; Sodium: 168mg; Carbohydrates: 27g; Fiber: 5g; Protein: 28g

Chicken *and* Wild Rice Soup

DAIRY-FREE, GLUTEN-FREE

Chicken and wild rice soup is a cozy lunch to have on a cold or rainy day. Soup can be a labor of love to make, but this recipe uses a slow cooker to make the cooking process seamless and easy! This soup achieves its creamy flavor with the help of full-fat coconut milk. **SERVES 8**

PREP TIME: 15 MINUTES
COOK TIME: 4 TO 8 HOURS

1 cup wild rice, rinsed and drained

1½ pounds boneless, skinless chicken breasts, chopped

4 cups chicken broth

1 cup diced carrots

1 cup diced celery

1 (8-ounce) package mushrooms, sliced

1 onion, diced

3 garlic cloves, minced

2 bay leaves

½ teaspoon dried thyme

½ teaspoon dried rosemary

½ cup full-fat coconut milk

¼ cup avocado oil or coconut oil

Fine sea salt

Freshly ground black pepper

Fresh thyme, for garnish

1.   In a slow cooker, combine the rice, chicken, chicken broth, carrots, celery, mushrooms, onion, garlic, bay leaves, thyme, and rosemary and mix well.

2.   Cover and cook on low for 8 hours or on high for 4 hours, until the chicken is completely cooked and the vegetables are soft.

3.   Add the coconut milk and avocado oil to the soup while it is still hot (but not cooking). Mix thoroughly. Season with salt and pepper to taste.

4.   Garnish with fresh thyme and serve, or store in a thermos to bring to work or school for lunch.

Cooking Tip: The amount of time it will take to make this soup (and several of the other recipes in this chapter and the Delicious Dinners chapter) will depend on the type of slow cooker you use. Check on the chicken just before the timer goes off, and add more time if needed.

Per Serving (2 cups or 1 bowl) Calories: 281; Total Fat: 12g; Saturated Fat: 9g; Sodium: 464mg; Carbohydrates: 21g; Fiber: 3g; Protein: 25g

Hearty Vegetable Soup

DAIRY-FREE, GLUTEN-FREE, VEGETARIAN, VEGAN

This soup may be meatless, but it is very hearty and satisfying! It is full of vegetables and minestrone-style Italian flavor. I think this recipe is especially appealing for lunch on chilly fall and winter days. **SERVES 4 TO 6**

PREP TIME: 15 MINUTES
COOK TIME: 45 MINUTES

3 tablespoons olive oil

1 medium yellow onion, chopped

3 carrots, peeled and chopped

2 celery stalks, chopped

1 cup chopped vegetable of choice (such as zucchini or butternut squash)

Fine sea salt

6 garlic cloves, minced

1 teaspoon dried thyme

1 (15-ounce) can diced tomatoes

½ cup low-sodium vegetable broth

2 cups filtered water

½ cup uncooked quinoa, rinsed well

2 bay leaves

1 (15-ounce) can chickpeas, rinsed and drained

1 cup chopped collard greens or kale

Freshly ground black pepper

1. Heat the olive oil in a soup pot over medium heat. Once the oil is simmering, add the onion, carrots, celery, squash (or vegetable of choice), and a pinch of salt and cook until the vegetables are soft.

2. Add the garlic, thyme, and diced tomatoes to the vegetable mixture in the pot. Cook for about 5 minutes.

3. Pour in the vegetable broth, water, and quinoa. Add 1 teaspoon of salt and the bay leaves. Raise the heat to a boil, cover the pot, reduce the heat to a simmer, and cook for 25 minutes.

4. Add the chickpeas and greens. Cook for 5 more minutes.

5. Remove the pot from the heat and season with salt and pepper to taste. Cool slightly before serving. Store this soup in the refrigerator for up to 1 week and in the freezer for up to 6 months.

Per Serving (1 bowl) Calories: 390; Total Fat: 14g; Saturated Fat: 2g; Sodium: 100mg; Carbohydrates: 56g; Fiber: 13g; Protein: 14g

Butternut Squash Chili

DAIRY-FREE, GLUTEN-FREE

This modern take on chili replaces beans with butternut squash, creating a nutritious, thick chili that doesn't skimp on flavor! Make a big batch on the weekend and enjoy for lunches (and dinners) throughout the week. **SERVES 8**

PREP TIME: 15 MINUTES
COOK TIME: 1 HOUR

2 tablespoons avocado oil or olive oil

1 yellow onion, chopped

4 garlic cloves, minced

1 pound ground beef (or bison)

1 pound ground pork

2 teaspoons onion powder

2 teaspoons garlic powder

2 teaspoons ground cumin

2 teaspoons paprika

2 teaspoons red pepper flakes

Fine sea salt

Freshly ground black pepper

1 cup chopped red bell pepper

1 small butternut squash, peeled and cubed

2 cups diced tomatoes, undrained

1 cup tomato sauce

1 cup low-sodium beef or chicken broth

1. In a large Dutch oven or enameled cast-iron soup pot, heat the avocado oil over medium heat. Add the onion and sauté for a few minutes. Add the garlic and continue to sauté until the onions are translucent and the garlic is tender.

2. Add the ground beef and pork and cook for about 5 minutes, breaking it up with a spoon.

3. Add the onion powder, garlic powder, cumin, paprika, red pepper flakes, salt, and pepper. Mix well.

4. Add the bell pepper, butternut squash, diced tomatoes with their juices, tomato sauce, and broth.

5. Stir the mixture, bring to a boil, cover the pot with a lid, and reduce to a simmer. Cook the chili for 30 to 40 minutes. Slightly cool before serving.

Make It a Meal: Serve the chili with a side salad and baked plantains for a complete south-of-the-border meal.

Per Serving (1 bowl) Calories: 286; Total Fat: 16g; Saturated Fat: 5g; Sodium: 258mg; Carbohydrates: 14g; Fiber: 3g; Protein: 23g

Cold Asian Zucchini Noodles *with* Chicken

DAIRY-FREE, GLUTEN-FREE, UNDER 30 MINUTES

This creamy chilled salad is perfect for satisfying a hankering for Asian food, but without the MSG and other unhealthy additives commonly found in Asian takeout and restaurant food. To make the zucchini noodles in this recipe, you will need a spiralizer or a julienne vegetable peeler. Both kitchen implements can be found online or in the kitchen section of your local home goods store. **SERVES 4**

PREP TIME: 15 MINUTES

FOR THE SALAD

2 large zucchini, washed and ends trimmed off, cut into "noodles" using a spiralizer or julienne vegetable peeler

1 large carrot, washed and ends trimmed off, cut into "noodles"

½ cup thinly sliced red cabbage

½ cup sliced sugar snap peas

2 scallions, thinly sliced

¼ cup chopped fresh cilantro leaves

2 cooked chicken breasts, shredded

Sliced cashews, for garnish (optional)

FOR THE SAUCE

½ cup creamy, unsweetened cashew butter

3 tablespoons coconut aminos

2 tablespoons avocado oil

1 tablespoon sesame oil

1 tablespoon filtered water

1 garlic clove, minced

1 teaspoon peeled and grated fresh gingerroot

Juice of 1 lime

TO MAKE THE SALAD

1. Place the zucchini noodles in a large bowl.

2. Add the carrot, cabbage, peas, scallions, cilantro, and shredded chicken to the noodles. Toss gently to combine.

TO MAKE THE SAUCE

1. In a small bowl, whisk together the cashew butter, coconut aminos, avocado oil, sesame oil, water, garlic, ginger, and lime juice.

2. Toss the sauce with the salad and garnish with cashews, if desired.

Ingredient Tip: You'll notice coconut aminos in the ingredient lists of several recipes throughout this book. Coconut aminos is a dark, rich, salty, and slightly sweet sauce derived from coconut sap that resembles a light soy sauce. It is a perfect replacement for those avoiding soy and gluten, which are common dietary allergens.

Per Serving (1 bowl) Calories: 402; Total Fat: 29g; Saturated Fat: 5g; Sodium: 80mg; Carbohydrates: 21g; Fiber: 4g; Protein: 18g

BLT Egg Lettuce Wraps

DAIRY-FREE, GLUTEN-FREE, UNDER 30 MINUTES

The BLT sandwich is a lunch classic. In these BLT wraps, sandwich bread is replaced with lettuce "wraps" for a healthier take on the traditional recipe. Make a large batch of hardboiled eggs at the beginning of the week during a meal prep session, and you'll have enough eggs to use in this recipe and several of the other recipes in this chapter.

SERVES 4

PREP TIME: 25 MINUTES

6 hardboiled eggs, diced

3 strips bacon, chopped, plus more for garnish (optional)

⅓ cup sliced cherry tomatoes

¼ cup finely diced celery

3 tablespoons finely diced red onion

3 tablespoons finely diced green onion, plus more for garnish (optional)

⅓ cup Avocado Oil Mayonnaise (page 91)

Butter lettuce leaves

Fine sea salt

Freshly ground black pepper

1. In a large mixing bowl, combine the eggs, bacon, tomatoes, celery, red onion, green onion, and avocado oil mayonnaise. Stir to mix.

2. Scoop dollops of the egg salad into the butter lettuce leaves. Garnish with green onion and bits of chopped bacon, if desired. Season with salt and pepper to taste.

Per Serving (3 lettuce wraps) Calories: 315; Total Fat: 28g; Saturated Fat: 6g; Sodium: 564mg; Carbohydrates: 3g; Fiber: 1g; Protein: 14g

Curried Egg Salad

DAIRY-FREE, GLUTEN-FREE, UNDER 30 MINUTES, VEGETARIAN

This curried egg salad is a unique, flavorful take on the traditional version. Even if you aren't normally a fan of egg salad, I guarantee you'll have a newfound appreciation for it after trying this recipe! **SERVES 4**

PREP TIME: 15 MINUTES

⅓ cup **Avocado Oil Mayonnaise (page 91)**

1¼ teaspoons **curry powder**

¼ teaspoon **ground turmeric**

2 teaspoons **freshly squeezed lime juice**

Fine sea salt

Freshly ground black pepper

8 **hardboiled eggs, diced**

⅓ cup **shredded carrot**

2 **green onions, chopped**

¼ cup **minced celery**

2 tablespoons **chopped fresh cilantro**

¼ cup **chopped cashews**

¼ cup **unsweetened raisins**

Mixed greens or cucumber slices, for serving

1. In a large bowl, mix together the mayonnaise, curry powder, turmeric, lime juice, a pinch of salt, and a dash of pepper.

2. Add the eggs, carrot, scallions, celery, cilantro, cashews, and raisins to the bowl and mix gently.

3. Serve the egg salad on a bed of mixed greens or cucumber slices. Store egg salad in the refrigerator for up to 1 week.

Per Serving (1 cup) Calories: 341; Total Fat: 28g; Saturated Fat: 6g; Sodium: 286mg; Carbohydrates: 12g; Fiber: 2g; Protein: 13g

Avocado Oil Mayonnaise

Several of the recipes in this chapter call for mayonnaise. However, conventional mayonnaise is typically loaded with industrial seed oils, which are highly inflammatory and will work against you in your efforts to recover from Lyme disease. Instead, I recommend making your own healthy mayonnaise using this simple, wholesome recipe featuring avocado oil and fresh egg. It is rich in anti-inflammatory healthy fats, not to mention delicious! **SERVES 20**

PREP TIME: 2 MINUTES

1 large egg, at room temperature

1 teaspoon Dijon mustard

2 teaspoons apple cider vinegar or white vinegar

¼ teaspoon fine sea salt

1 cup avocado oil

1. Crack the egg into the bottom of a glass Mason jar. Add the Dijon mustard, vinegar, and salt on top of the egg. Do not whisk or stir.

2. Pour the avocado oil on top of the ingredients in the glass jar.

3. Submerge an immersion blender into the jar. Blend on low power for 20 seconds, or until the mixture has turned white and homogenous. Then, slowly move the blender up and down in the jar to evenly blend the mayo. Alternately, you can mix the mayonnaise with a whisk.

4. Store in a jar in the fridge for up to 1 week. I recommend making a fresh batch each week to use with the recipes in this chapter.

Per Serving (1 tablespoon) Calories: 100; Total Fat: 11g; Saturated Fat: 1g; Sodium: 14mg; Carbohydrates: 0g; Fiber: 0g; Protein: 0g

Turmeric Chickpea Cauliflower Rice

DAIRY-FREE, GLUTEN-FREE, VEGETARIAN, VEGAN

Buddha bowls, vegetarian meals served in single bowls consisting of small portions of several foods, are currently all the rage in the health world. This recipe, brimming with nutritious vegetables and Indian flavor, will help you understand why this food trend has become so popular. It is delicious and extremely easy to prepare, making it a lunch recipe you'll come back to again and again. **SERVES 4**

PREP TIME: 15 MINUTES
COOK TIME: 25 MINUTES

FOR THE CAULIFLOWER RICE

1 small head cauliflower, chopped, washed, and patted dry

1 teaspoon avocado oil

½ small yellow onion, minced

¼ teaspoon fine sea salt

1 teaspoon ground turmeric

Dash of freshly squeezed lemon or lime juice

FOR THE CHICKPEAS AND CARROTS

¼ teaspoon avocado oil

1 teaspoon ground cumin

1 teaspoon ground coriander

½ teaspoon paprika

½ teaspoon garlic powder

1 (15-ounce) can chickpeas, drained

¾ cup sliced carrots

Mixed greens, for serving

Freshly squeezed lemon juice (optional)

TO MAKE THE CAULIFLOWER RICE

1. Grate the cauliflower using a cheese grater or a food processor. (Using a food processor is MUCH easier, so I highly recommend getting one for your kitchen!)

2. Heat the avocado oil in a skillet over medium heat. Add the onions and a pinch of salt, cooking until the onions are translucent, about 5 to 7 minutes.

3. Add the turmeric to the onions, stir, and then add the riced cauliflower, lemon juice, and the remaining salt. Cover and cook for 6 to 8 minutes.

4. Remove from the heat and fluff the "rice."

TO MAKE THE CHICKPEAS AND CARROTS

1. In a separate skillet over low heat, heat the avocado oil, cumin, coriander, paprika, and garlic powder. Add the chickpeas, tossing and coating them in the oil. Cook for 1 minute, then add the carrots. Add 2 tablespoons of filtered water to the pan to soften the carrots. Cover and cook for 5 minutes, then set aside and let cool.

2. Make a bed of greens and top with the cauliflower rice and chickpea-carrot mixture. Drizzle lemon juice on top, if desired.

Per Serving (2 cups) Calories: 179; Total Fat: 4g; Saturated Fat: 1g; Sodium: 158mg; Carbohydrates: 30g; Fiber: 9g; Protein: 9g

Cashew Tuna Salad

DAIRY-FREE, GLUTEN-FREE, UNDER 30 MINUTES

Tuna salad—you either love it or hate it! After trying this recipe, I think you'll officially become a tuna salad lover! The cashews add an unexpected crunch and richness to this salad, turning a normally homogenous dish into a play on textures. **SERVES 4**

PREP TIME: 10 MINUTES

2 (5-ounce) cans tuna (preferably wild-caught), drained

½ cup broccoli slaw

½ cup diced yellow bell pepper

⅓ cup diced yellow onion

¼ cup chopped cashews

½ cup Avocado Oil Mayonnaise (page 91)

Juice of 1 lemon

¼ cup chopped fresh basil

Fine sea salt

Freshly ground black pepper

In a medium bowl, combine the tuna, broccoli slaw, bell pepper, onion, and cashews. Slowly add the mayonnaise—you may want less or more, depending on how creamy you like your tuna salad. Add the lemon juice and basil. Stir gently until you have a smooth mixture. Season with salt and pepper to taste.

Make It a Meal: Add the tuna salad to a bed of salad greens, or eat on top of cucumber slices or crackers.

Per Serving (1 cup) Calories: 376; Total Fat: 30g; Saturated Fat: 5g; Sodium: 223mg; Carbohydrates: 6g; Fiber: 1g; Protein: 21g

Sweet Potato Ramen Bowl

DAIRY-FREE, GLUTEN-FREE, UNDER 30 MINUTES, VEGETARIAN

Gourmet ramen is currently a trending dish in restaurants across the country—this isn't the packaged, microwavable ramen of your college days! For this ramen recipe, you'll need to pull out your spiralizer or julienne vegetable peeler to make the sweet potato ramen "noodles," which take the place of traditional grain-based noodles. The result is a more nutritious and colorful ramen that will delight your eyes and your taste buds! SERVES 2

PREP TIME: 10 MINUTES
COOK TIME: 10 MINUTES

2 large eggs

4 cups low-sodium vegetable broth or chicken broth

1½ teaspoons coconut aminos or organic gluten-free soy sauce

2 large sweet potatoes, peeled and spiralized or julienned

1 cup sliced red cabbage

1 cup shredded carrot

Fine sea salt

Freshly ground black pepper

Hot chili oil

2 green onions, chopped, for garnish

1. Make the softboiled eggs: Bring a pot of water to a boil then reduce to a rapid simmer. Add the eggs and cook for 5 minutes. This length of time will typically yield an egg with a soft yolk. Remove the eggs and allow them to cool before peeling.

2. In a soup pot, combine the broth and coconut aminos and bring to a boil. Add the sweet potato "noodles" and cook until soft, about 5 minutes.

3. Remove the soup from the heat and add the cabbage and carrot. You still want them to be slightly crunchy, so you don't want to cook them with the sweet potatoes.

4. If you want to include meat in this dish, add it now. Add salt and pepper to taste.

5. Ladle the soup into bowls, adding one softboiled egg each that has been cut in half. Drizzle with hot chili oil and garnish with green onions.

Cooking Tip: Add chicken, beef, or pork to this recipe for more protein, if desired.

Per Serving (1 bowl with 1 egg) Calories: 298; Total Fat: 8g; Saturated Fat: 2g; Sodium: 452mg; Carbohydrates: 37g; Fiber: 7g; Protein: 20g

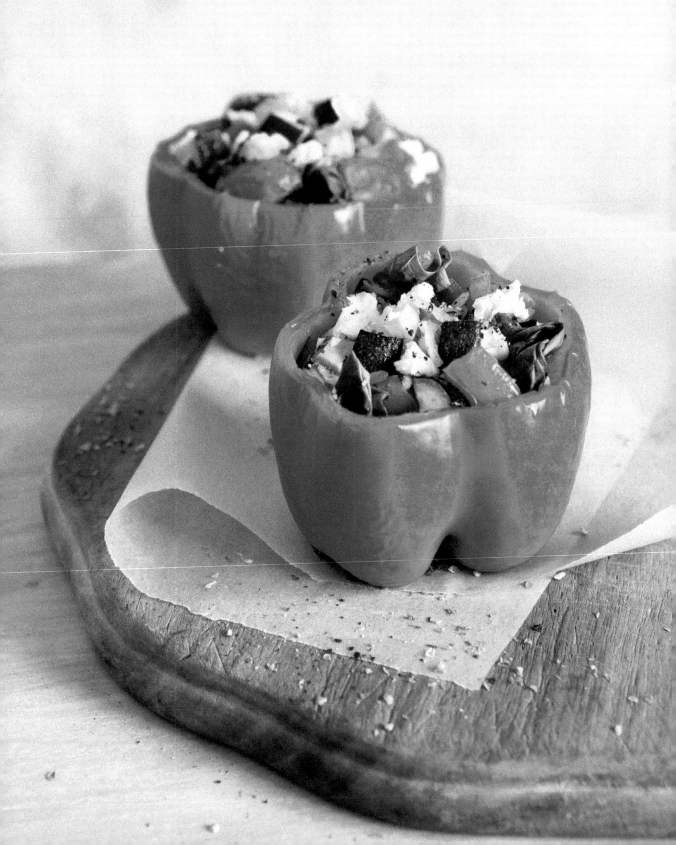

Chapter 6

Delicious Dinners

Energize your body and mind with meals that are as flavorful as they are nutritious. All of the recipes in this chapter feature loads of vegetables and healthy proteins and fats that will fill you up without weighing you down or leaving you feeling drained at the end of the day. Whether you're in the mood for comfort food, international flavors, or something a little sophisticated, you'll find it here. And the best part? Each dish is simple to prepare, requiring easy-to-find ingredients and very little intensive prep and cooking work.

Chinese Chicken Salad
with Cauliflower Rice

DAIRY-FREE, GLUTEN-FREE

Chinese takeout is a go-to dinner for many people. However, the typical Chinese take-out menu is a sea of nutritional no-nos, including deep-fried dishes, fake seafood, and MSG. This fresh, delicious chicken salad is the perfect healthy alternative. Shredded cabbage makes it delightfully crunchy, and mandarin orange slices add just a touch of sweetness. This is a recipe my nutrition clients come to again and again, and I think you will, too! SERVES 4

PREP TIME: 15 MINUTES
COOK TIME: 25 MINUTES

FOR THE SALAD

2 (6-ounce) boneless, skinless
  chicken breasts

1 tablespoon avocado oil

½ teaspoon fine sea salt

½ teaspoon freshly ground black pepper

1 head iceberg or romaine lettuce, cored
  and sliced

¼ head red cabbage, sliced

1 bell pepper (any color), seeded and sliced

6 green onions, sliced

4 sprigs fresh cilantro, finely chopped

2 (10-ounce) cans unsweetened mandarin
  oranges, drained

1 cup roasted and sliced almonds
  or cashews

FOR THE DRESSING

¼ cup avocado oil

¼ cup rice wine vinegar

3 tablespoons organic gluten-free soy
  sauce or coconut aminos

2 pitted dates

2 teaspoons sesame oil

½ teaspoon fine sea salt

TO MAKE THE SALAD AND DRESSING

1. Preheat the oven to 375°F. Line a baking sheet with parchment paper.

2. Lay the chicken breasts on the parchment paper and drizzle with avocado oil, salt, and pepper. Roast in the oven for 20 minutes, or until the chicken has reached an internal temperature of 165°F and is cooked all the way through. Remove the cooked chicken from the oven and cut into bite-size pieces.

3. Combine the dressing ingredients in a blender or food processor. Blend until smooth.

4. In a large bowl, combine the lettuce, cabbage, bell pepper, green onion, cilantro, mandarin oranges, and nuts. Toss gently to mix. Add the chicken and dressing.

FOR THE CAULIFLOWER "RICE"

4 cups chopped cauliflower florets

2 tablespoons sesame oil

Fine sea salt

Freshly ground black pepper

TO MAKE THE CAULIFLOWER "RICE"

1. Cut the cauliflower into florets. Add the florets to a food processor three at a time so as not to overwhelm the food processor's capabilities! On the stovetop over medium heat, coat a skillet with 1 to 2 tablespoons of sesame oil. When it is hot, add the riced cauliflower and a dash of salt and pepper to taste. Cook for 3 to 4 minutes until the cauliflower has softened. Remove from the heat.

2. Garnish the rice with chopped green onion and serve alongside the salad. This meal also tastes great cold as lunch the next day!

Per Serving (1 cup chicken salad with 1 cup cauliflower "rice") Calories: 655; Total Fat: 44g; Saturated Fat: 5g; Sodium: 567mg; Carbohydrates: 41g; Fiber: 10g; Protein: 31g

Beef *and* Veggie Stir-Fry

DAIRY-FREE, GLUTEN-FREE, UNDER 30 MINUTES, VEGAN OPTION

Stir-fries are a great way to make nutritious meals from all those leftover ingredients hanging out in your fridge. This recipe primarily uses broccoli, but feel free to try cauliflower, carrots, and bell pepper, too. **SERVES 3**

PREP TIME: 10 MINUTES
COOK TIME: 15 TO 20 MINUTES

¾ cup organic gluten-free soy sauce or coconut aminos

1 tablespoon toasted sesame oil

3 tablespoons freshly squeezed lemon or lime juice

3 garlic cloves, minced

1 inch fresh gingerroot, peeled and minced

½ teaspoon red pepper flakes

Fine sea salt

Freshly ground black pepper

1 pound flank steak, thinly sliced

Avocado oil

Florets from 2 heads broccoli

Water chestnuts, chopped green onions, sesame seeds (optional)

1. In a small bowl or food processor, combine the soy sauce, sesame oil, lemon juice, garlic, ginger, red pepper flakes, a pinch of salt, and a dash of pepper to make the sauce. Using a food processor will yield a smoother sauce.

2. Season the sliced steak with salt and pepper. Heat a large pan over medium heat and pour in enough avocado oil to coat it and prevent the steak from sticking. Add slices of beef, cooking about 30 seconds on each side.

3. Once the beef is cooked, remove it from the pan and set aside. Leaving the beef juices in the pan, add the broccoli florets. Add 3 tablespoons of sauce and cook until the broccoli is tender, about 5 to 10 minutes.

4. Add the beef and remaining sauce back to the pan. Reduce the heat to low and cook until the sauce is thickened, about 2 to 3 minutes. Add the water chestnuts, green onions, and sesame seeds (if using).

5. Remove the pan from the heat and allow to cool before serving.

Substitution Tip: Make this meal vegan/vegetarian by subbing organic tofu or tempeh for the beef. Or, alternatively, use whatever meat you have on hand for this recipe—sliced chicken and turkey breast work just as well as beef.

Make It a Meal: Serve this stir-fry with a side of brown rice or cauliflower rice.

Per Serving (1 bowl) Calories: 410; Total Fat: 17g; Saturated Fat: 1g; Sodium: 229mg; Carbohydrates: 30g; Fiber: 7g; Protein: 36g

Grain-Free Shepherd's Pie

DAIRY-FREE, GLUTEN-FREE

Shepherd's pie is the quintessential comfort food. Thick, creamy, and filling, it will make you feel cozy and content at the end of a long day. Traditional shepherd's pie uses refined flour to make the crust and white potatoes and heavy cream in the filling; this recipe eschews refined flour and dairy and uses nutritious sweet potatoes in the topping. SERVES 8

PREP TIME: 20 MINUTES
COOK TIME: 1 HOUR

FOR THE SWEET POTATO TOPPING

4 sweet potatoes (2½ pounds), peeled and chopped into 2-inch pieces

⅔ cup full-fat coconut milk

3 tablespoons avocado oil

3 tablespoons nutritional yeast (this adds a savory flavor; omit if you are sensitive to yeast)

Fine sea salt

Freshly ground black pepper

FOR THE BEEF AND VEGETABLE FILLING

1 tablespoon avocado oil

1½ pounds ground beef

Fine sea salt

1 teaspoon chopped fresh thyme

1 teaspoon chopped fresh rosemary

¾ cup low-sodium beef bone broth

1 cup chopped Brussels sprouts

1 cup diced carrots

1 onion, chopped

1 cup chopped mushrooms

2 garlic cloves, minced

Freshly ground black pepper

TO MAKE THE SWEET POTATO TOPPING

1. Fill a large stockpot with filtered water and bring to a boil. Add the sweet potato pieces and cook until very soft.

2. Drain the potatoes, add the coconut milk and avocado oil, and mash with a potato masher until smooth. Mix in the nutritional yeast and add salt and pepper to taste. You can also use an immersion blender to make extra-smooth mashed sweet potatoes.

TO MAKE THE BEEF AND VEGETABLE FILLING AND BAKE THE PIE

1. In a cast-iron or other ovenproof skillet, add the avocado oil, ground beef, and a dash of salt and brown evenly. Break up any lumps with a wooden spoon. Add the thyme, rosemary, and broth and simmer to let the broth reduce. Remove from the skillet and set aside.

2. Add the Brussels sprouts, carrots, onion, and mushrooms to the skillet. After 2 minutes, add the garlic, and salt and pepper to taste. Cook until all vegetables are fork-tender.

3. Preheat the oven to 375°F. →

4. Once the vegetables are cooked, return the ground beef to the skillet, stirring to combine. Top with the mashed sweet potatoes. Spread the mashed potatoes evenly over the beef and veggie mixture.

5. Bake the pie for 20 minutes, or until the sweet potatoes are a light golden brown on top. Allow to cool for 10 minutes before serving. Store any leftovers in the refrigerator for up to 1 week or in the freezer for up to 6 months.

Per Serving (1 slice) Calories: 354; Total Fat: 12g; Saturated Fat: 7g; Sodium: 189mg; Carbohydrates: 44g; Fiber: 7g; Protein: 23g

Spaghetti Squash "Pasta" *with* Meatballs *and* Marinara Sauce

DAIRY-FREE, GLUTEN-FREE

Do you love the taste of spaghetti but hate the "carb coma" that comes after eating a heaping plate of pasta? If you answered yes, then this recipe is for you! Spaghetti squash makes for a lighter, more nutritious alternative to grain-based pasta. It will leave your taste buds tingling with Italian flavors, sans carb coma! SERVES 4

PREP TIME: 20 MINUTES
COOK TIME: 50 MINUTES

FOR THE SQUASH "SPAGHETTI"

1 tablespoon olive oil, divided

1 large spaghetti squash, halved and deseeded

Fine sea salt

FOR THE MARINARA SAUCE

3 tablespoons olive oil, divided

½ yellow onion, finely diced

Fine sea salt

2 garlic cloves, minced

3 tablespoons tomato paste

1 (28-ounce) can crushed tomatoes

2 tablespoons chopped fresh parsley

FOR THE MEATBALLS

1 pound ground beef

1 pound ground pork

½ onion, chopped

½ cup fresh parsley, loosely packed

2 garlic cloves, crushed

½ teaspoon dried basil

½ teaspoon dried oregano

1 egg yolk

2 tablespoons olive oil

TO MAKE THE SQUASH "SPAGHETTI"

1. Preheat the oven to 400°F. Line a baking sheet with parchment paper and drizzle olive oil on top.

2. Place the squash halves face-down on the prepared baking sheet and slide around to coat with olive oil. Bake for 30 to 40 minutes until the squash is tender and comes apart in spaghetti-like strands.

TO MAKE THE MARINARA SAUCE

1. Place a saucepan over medium-high heat and pour in 1 tablespoon of olive oil. Once the olive oil is heated, add the onion and a dash of salt and cook for about 2 minutes until the onion is translucent.

2. Add the garlic and tomato paste and cook for 1 minute. Add the crushed tomatoes and the remaining 2 tablespoons of olive oil, bring to a boil, and then reduce to medium-low heat. Cover and simmer for 25 to 30 minutes. →

TO MAKE THE MEATBALLS

1.   In a food processor, combine the beef, pork, onion, parsley, garlic, basil, oregano, and egg yolk and mix until smooth. Form the mixture into meatballs the size of ping-pong balls.

2.   In a large skillet over medium heat, heat enough olive oil to coat the pan, bringing it to a simmer. Cook the meatballs until they are browned on all sides and cooked through, about 15 minutes.

3.   Shred the spaghetti squash into "noodles," portion into bowls, and season with salt to taste. Top with the marinara sauce and meatballs. Garnish with fresh parsley.

Make It a Meal: To fit extra veggies into this meal, try mixing broccoli or cauliflower with the marinara sauce, or make a side salad to accompany your "spaghetti."

Per Serving (1 bowl) Calories: 644; Total Fat: 40g; Saturated Fat: 9g; Sodium: 627mg; Carbohydrates: 30g; Fiber: 8g; Protein: 52g

Balsamic Chicken *with* Brussels Sprouts *and* Bacon

DAIRY-FREE, GLUTEN-FREE

Sheet-pan meals are a convenient way to quickly throw together a delicious, healthy dinner. This recipe levels up classic baked chicken and Brussels sprouts by adding savory balsamic vinegar and smoky bacon. You'll want to marinate the chicken for at least 5 minutes; to get the most flavorful chicken, I recommend marinating it overnight for 12 hours. SERVES 4

PREP TIME: 10 MINUTES
COOK TIME: 25 MINUTES

- ¼ cup balsamic vinegar
- ⅓ cup olive oil
- Juice of ½ lemon
- 2 garlic cloves, crushed
- ¼ cup finely chopped fresh rosemary
- 2 (6-ounce) boneless, skinless chicken breasts, halved
- 10 ounces Brussels sprouts, stemmed and halved
- 6 low-sodium bacon slices, chopped
- Fine sea salt
- Freshly ground black pepper

1. In a blender or food processor, combine the vinegar, olive oil, lemon juice, and garlic. Pulse to combine. Add the rosemary and blend again. Place the chicken breasts in a glass dish and pour the marinade on top. Let the meat marinate for anywhere from 5 minutes to 12 hours.

2. Preheat the oven to 375°F. Line a large sheet pan with parchment paper or aluminum foil.

3. Place the marinated chicken, Brussels sprouts, and bacon on the sheet pan and cover with the remaining marinade. Use a marinade brush to evenly coat the ingredients.

4. Bake until the juices of the chicken breasts run clear or the breasts reach an internal temperature of 165°F.

5. Remove from the oven. Add salt and pepper to taste and serve.

Per Serving (½ chicken breast with 1 cup Brussels sprouts and bacon) Calories: 285; Total Fat: 13g; Saturated Fat: 4g; Sodium: 397mg; Carbohydrates: 8g; Fiber: 3g; Protein: 32g

Burgers *and* Sweet Potato Fries

DAIRY-FREE, GLUTEN-FREE

These burgers are super easy to make and full of flavor! Sweet potato fries offer a more nutritious alternative to traditional fries made with regular potatoes. Top your burger with tomato, onion, and avocado to load up on veggies. **SERVES 6**

PREP TIME: 10 MINUTES
COOK TIME: 30 MINUTES

FOR THE SWEET POTATO FRIES

4 large sweet potatoes

2 tablespoons avocado oil

Fine sea salt

Chipotle powder, for seasoning (optional)

FOR THE BURGERS

1½ pounds lean ground beef

1 teaspoon garlic powder

1 teaspoon freshly ground black pepper

1 teaspoon fine sea salt

1 tablespoon avocado oil

TO MAKE THE SWEET POTATO FRIES

1. Preheat the oven to 450°F. Line a baking sheet with parchment paper and set aside.

2. Peel the sweet potatoes, cut off the ends, and cut lengthwise into fry-shaped sticks. Put the sweet potatoes into a large bowl, add the avocado oil, and toss to coat. Add a dash of salt. You can also add spices such as chipotle powder, if you like.

3. Spread the sweet potatoes in a single layer on a baking sheet lined with parchment paper. Bake for 25 to 30 minutes, or until the fries are crisp.

TO MAKE THE BURGERS

1. Mix the ground beef, garlic powder, pepper, and salt thoroughly in a large bowl. Shape into 6 patties.

2. Heat a large skillet over medium heat. Pour in 1 tablespoon of avocado oil to prevent the burgers from sticking.

3. Place the burgers in the skillet and sauté for 3 to 5 minutes on each side. Reduce the heat to low and cover the skillet with the lid. Cook the burgers for 5 to 6 more minutes, or until they are cooked all the way through.

4. Allow the burgers to cool for a couple minutes before eating.

Serving Tips: Serve these burgers on whole-grain or gluten-free buns or a bed of salad greens, with your favorite toppings. Pair the sweet potato fries with a no-sugar-added ketchup.

Per Serving (1 burger with 12 fries [about 3 ounces of fries]) Calories: 278; Total Fat: 13g; Saturated Fat: 4g; Sodium: 445mg; Carbohydrates: 18g; Fiber: 3g; Protein: 24g

Zucchini Noodles *with* Peas

DAIRY-FREE, GLUTEN-FREE, UNDER 30 MINUTES, VEGETARIAN, VEGAN

It's time to get out your spiralizer again to make this refreshing dinner that's perfect for warm spring and summer nights. This recipe makes use of fresh, seasonal ingredients including zucchini, peas, and mint leaves. It also tastes wonderful chilled the next day for lunch! **SERVES 6**

PREP TIME: 10 MINUTES
COOK TIME: 15 MINUTES

5 tablespoons extra-virgin olive oil, divided

1 shallot, minced

3 cups shelled peas, fresh or frozen

6 garlic cloves, minced

6 zucchini, spiralized into noodles

Juice of 1 lemon

Zest of 1 lemon

Fine sea salt

⅛ teaspoon freshly ground black pepper

¼ cup fresh mint leaves, chopped

1. In a large pot over medium-high heat, bring 3 tablespoons of olive oil to a simmer.

2. Add the shallot. Cook for about 5 minutes, until soft.

3. Add the peas. Cook for 4 minutes, stirring occasionally.

4. Add the garlic and cook for 30 seconds, stirring the entire time.

5. Add the zucchini noodles, lemon juice and zest, a dash of salt, and pepper. Cook for 4 to 5 minutes, until the noodles are al dente.

6. Toss the noodles with the remaining 2 tablespoons of olive oil and the mint leaves before serving.

Cooking Tip: If you don't have a spiralizer, use a vegetable peeler to peel the zucchini into ribbons.

Per Serving (1 cup) Calories: 199; Total Fat: 12g; Saturated Fat: 2g; Sodium: 27mg; Carbohydrates: 19g; Fiber: 6g; Protein: 7g

Slow Cooker Sloppy Joes

DAIRY-FREE, GLUTEN-FREE OPTION

When I was growing up in Illinois, sloppy joes were a recurring item on my family's dinner menu. Even as an adult, I feel a certain nostalgia when I have sloppy joes— maybe it's a Midwest thing! This recipe uses wholesome ingredients to create a healthy update of this cozy, comforting classic. **SERVES 6**

PREP TIME: 10 MINUTES
COOK TIME: 8 HOURS

½ large onion, finely diced

1 bell pepper (any color), seeded and finely diced

1½ pounds lean ground beef (or ground bison or turkey), broken up into small pieces

16 ounces tomato paste

3 tablespoons apple cider vinegar

2 tablespoons pure maple syrup

1 tablespoon coconut aminos or organic gluten-free soy sauce

2 teaspoons Dijon mustard

1 teaspoon garlic powder

1 cup filtered water

1 teaspoon fine sea salt

Freshly ground black pepper

Whole-grain buns, for serving (optional)

1. In a slow cooker, combine the onion, bell pepper, ground beef, tomato paste, vinegar, maple syrup, coconut aminos, Dijon mustard, garlic powder, and water. Cover and cook for 4 hours on high or 8 hours on low. Stir the meat occasionally to break it up into small chunks. Add the salt and season with pepper to taste.

2. Once the meat is done, serve the sloppy joes on buns, if you like.

Substitution Tips: To make this meal gluten-free, serve the sloppy joes on gluten-free buns rather than whole-grain buns. If you are avoiding grains altogether, pair the sloppy joes with baked sweet potatoes and a side salad.

Per Serving (1 sandwich) Calories: 256; Total Fat: 9g; Saturated Fat: 3g; Sodium: 643mg; Carbohydrates: 22g; Fiber: 4g; Protein: 26g

Slow Cooker Chicken Tacos

DAIRY-FREE, GLUTEN-FREE OPTION

Tacos are an excellent "build-your-own" meal that is fun for the whole family and appropriate on Taco Tuesday or any other night of the week! This recipe uses a slow cooker to make taco meat that is extra tender and flavorful. **SERVES 4**

PREP TIME: 10 MINUTES
COOK TIME: 4 HOURS 30 MINUTES TO
5 HOURS 30 MINUTES

1 pound boneless, skinless chicken breast

1 pound boneless, skinless chicken thighs

½ cup filtered water

1 cup salsa, plus more for serving (optional)

1 teaspoon garlic powder

2 teaspoons chili powder

2 teaspoons ground cumin

¼ teaspoon cayenne pepper

Fine sea salt

Freshly ground black pepper

Tortillas, for serving (optional)

Lettuce or greens, for serving (optional)

Guacamole or sliced avocado, for serving (optional)

1. In a slow cooker, combine the chicken breasts and thighs, water, salsa, garlic powder, chili powder, cumin, and cayenne. Cover and cook on high for 4 to 5 hours.

2. Remove the chicken, place on a plate, and shred with a fork. Return the meat to the slow cooker and cook for another 30 minutes. Season with salt and pepper to taste.

3. Scoop the taco meat onto tortillas, lettuce leaves (which you can use as wraps), or atop a bed of greens. Top with salsa, guacamole, or avocado slices, if desired.

Substitution Tip: You can make this recipe gluten-free by subbing corn tortillas or cassava flour tortillas (such as Siete grain-free tortillas) for traditional flour tortillas.

Per Serving (2 tacos) Calories: 288; Total Fat: 8g; Saturated Fat: 1g; Sodium: 621mg; Carbohydrates: 6g; Fiber: 2g; Protein: 48g

Red Lentil Dal

DAIRY-FREE, GLUTEN-FREE, VEGETARIAN, VEGAN

Dal is a traditional Indian dish that uses dried, split legumes to make thick, hearty stews. This dal, made with red lentils, is rich in color and flavor. Lentils are an excellent source of prebiotic fiber, which feeds the beneficial bacteria in your gut and has anti-inflammatory effects. Though dal often contains dairy, this recipe uses full-fat coconut milk instead to achieve a thick, creamy consistency. **SERVES 4**

PREP TIME: 10 MINUTES
COOK TIME: 30 MINUTES

2 tablespoons melted coconut oil

1 onion, diced

1 tablespoon peeled and grated fresh gingerroot

1 tomato, finely chopped

1 red chile, seeded and finely chopped

Fine sea salt

2 teaspoons ground cumin

1 teaspoon mustard seeds

1 teaspoon ground coriander

1 teaspoon ground cinnamon

1 teaspoon ground turmeric

2 garlic cloves, minced

1 cup uncooked red lentils, rinsed and drained

3 cups vegetable broth

1 cup full-fat coconut milk

Juice of 1 lemon

Freshly ground black pepper

1. In a large soup pot over medium heat, combine the coconut oil, onion, ginger, tomato, and chile. Add a dash of salt and cook for 5 minutes, until the onions are fragrant and translucent, stirring occasionally.

2. Add the cumin, mustard seeds, coriander, cinnamon, turmeric, and garlic. Cook until fragrant. Add the lentils, broth, and coconut milk. When the mixture starts bubbling, reduce the heat to low.

3. Cook the dal on low for 20 minutes, or until the lentils become very soft and creamy.

4. Remove from heat and add the lemon juice. Season with pepper to taste. Let cool before serving.

Make It a Meal: Serve this dal alongside brown rice or cauliflower rice or roti, a traditional Indian flatbread.

Ingredient Tip: Enhance the nutritional benefits of lentils by soaking them before cooking. The soaking process reduces levels of antinutrients, such as phytates and lectins, which interfere with nutrient absorption and digestion. To properly soak lentils, follow these simple steps:

1. Pour your lentils in a large pot and cover with cold, filtered water. Let the lentils soak for 2 to 4 hours.

2. Drain the lentils and rinse them briefly under cold, filtered water. The lentils are now ready to be cooked.

Per Serving (1 cup) Calories: 392; Total Fat: 22g; Saturated Fat: 19g; Sodium: 75mg; Carbohydrates: 37g; Fiber: 17g; Protein: 15g

Lemon-Garlic Salmon

Wild-caught seafood is, hands down, the best dietary source of omega-3 fatty acids. Omega-3s are essential for maintaining a healthy brain and inflammatory balance in the body. I recommend eating wild-caught seafood, such as the salmon used in this recipe, two to three times a week to optimize your omega-3 level. After tasting this recipe, you'll realize just how easy and delicious it is to add seafood to your diet!

SERVES 4

PREP TIME: 10 MINUTES
COOK TIME: 15 MINUTES

¼ cup ghee

6 to 8 garlic cloves, minced

¼ cup low-sodium fish broth or chicken broth

¼ cup freshly squeezed lemon juice

Fine sea salt

4 (6-ounce) wild-caught salmon fillets

Freshly ground black pepper

1 tablespoon avocado oil

Chopped fresh parsley, for garnish

1. In a saucepan, melt the ghee over medium heat. Add the garlic and sauté until fragrant.

2. Add the broth, lemon juice, and salt. Simmer until the mixture is reduced by half. Remove from the heat and set aside.

3. Season the salmon fillets with salt and pepper on both sides. Heat the avocado oil in a saucepan over medium heat until the oil is simmering.

4. Gently place the fillets in the pan skin-side up and cook until lightly browned on the bottom, about 2 to 3 minutes. Use a spatula to gently flip the fish and cook for 3 to 4 minutes on the other side (the side with the skin).

5. Remove the salmon from the heat and cover with the lemon-garlic sauce. Garnish with fresh parsley and serve.

Make It a Meal: Serve this salmon with a fresh salad and wild rice.

Ingredient Tip: Ghee is derived from milk, but it goes through an extensive filtration process that eliminates essentially all milk proteins. As a result, it is a highly nutritious, anti-inflammatory, and delicious cooking fat that makes a perfect substitute for butter.

Per Serving (1 fillet) Calories: 530; Total Fat: 43g; Saturated Fat: 15g; Sodium: 195mg; Carbohydrates: 5g; Fiber: 1g; Protein: 32g

Simple Fish Curry

DAIRY-FREE, GLUTEN-FREE, UNDER 30 MINUTES

This fish curry is loaded with anti-inflammatory ingredients and amazing Thai flavor. Ginger and turmeric are superfoods that reduce joint pain and heal the gut, and fish provides an abundance of anti-inflammatory omega-3 fatty acids. **SERVES 2**

PREP TIME: 15 MINUTES
COOK TIME: 15 MINUTES

1 tablespoon coconut oil

1 red onion, finely chopped

2 teaspoons peeled and grated fresh gingerroot

2 garlic cloves, crushed

1 teaspoon ground turmeric

¼ teaspoon ground cumin

½ teaspoon red pepper flakes

1 (14-ounce) can full-fat coconut milk

Freshly squeezed juice of ½ lime

Fine sea salt

Freshly ground black pepper

2 (8-ounce) white fish fillets, such as snapper

Chopped fresh cilantro, for garnishing (optional)

1. Melt the coconut oil in a large pan over medium-high heat. Add the onion and cook until fragrant and translucent.

2. Add the ginger, garlic, turmeric, cumin, and red pepper flakes. Stir for about 1 minute.

3. Add the coconut milk, lime juice, and a dash of salt and pepper. Mix thoroughly.

4. Add the fish and cook for 10 minutes, or until the fish flakes easily.

5. Remove the fish from the heat and garnish with fresh cilantro (if using).

Make It a Meal: Serve this curry with basmati rice or cauliflower rice for a complete meal.

Per Serving (1 fillet with ½ cup of sauce)
Calories: 851; Total Fat: 59g; Saturated Fat: 48g; Sodium: 192mg; Carbohydrates: 20g; Fiber: 6g; Protein: 65g

Stuffed Bell Peppers

DAIRY-FREE, GLUTEN-FREE, VEGETARIAN, VEGAN

Looking for a Mexican food-inspired dish but not in the mood for a heavy taco or burrito? Look no further than these stuffed bell peppers. Bursting with south-of-the-border flavor, these peppers are spicy and filling, not to mention gluten-free and vegan!

SERVES 4

PREP TIME: 10 MINUTES
COOK TIME: 1 HOUR

1 cup uncooked quinoa, rinsed and drained

2 cups vegetable broth

Avocado oil, for greasing

4 large bell peppers, seeded and halved

1 (15-ounce) can black beans, rinsed and drained

½ cup salsa

2 teaspoons ground cumin

1½ teaspoons chili powder

1½ teaspoons garlic powder

Fine sea salt

Freshly ground black pepper

Guacamole or sliced avocado, for serving (optional)

Hot sauce, for serving (optional)

Freshly squeezed lime juice, for serving (optional)

1. Combine the quinoa and vegetable broth in a saucepan and bring to a boil over high heat. Once it is boiling, reduce the heat and simmer until all the liquid has been absorbed and the quinoa is fluffy, about 20 minutes.

2. Preheat the oven to 375°F and lightly grease a baking sheet with avocado oil. Alternatively, you can line the sheet with parchment paper.

3. Brush the halved peppers with a light layer of avocado oil.

4. In a large mixing bowl, mix the quinoa, black beans, salsa, cumin, chili powder, and garlic powder. Add salt and pepper to taste.

5. Stuff the halved peppers with the quinoa–black bean mixture and place them on the prepared baking sheet. Cover the sheet with aluminum foil. If you are using a Dutch oven, put the lid on the dish. Bake for 30 minutes covered. After 30 minutes, remove the foil or lid and bake for 10 more minutes. The peppers should end up soft and a light golden brown.

6. Let cool for 5 minutes before serving. Top with guacamole or avocado slices, hot sauce, or lime juice, if desired.

Substitution Tip: Don't need this recipe to be vegetarian? Swap the quinoa for ground beef or turkey.

Per Serving (1 stuffed pepper) Calories: 327; Total Fat: 4g; Saturated Fat: 1g; Sodium: 272mg; Carbohydrates: 61g; Fiber: 13g; Protein: 16g

Kale, Lamb, *and* Sweet Potato Soup

GLUTEN-FREE

This one-pot meal is cozy, comforting, and loaded with nutritious lamb and vegetables. Choose grass-fed, organic lamb to maximize the nutritional quality of this dish, as the meat of grass-fed animals is higher in omega-3 fatty acids and antioxidants than meat from grain-fed animals. SERVES 4

PREP TIME: 15 MINUTES
COOK TIME: 55 MINUTES

1 pound boneless lamb shoulder, cut into 1-inch pieces

2 tablespoons tapioca flour

1 tablespoon ghee or avocado oil

1 medium sweet onion, diced

2 garlic cloves, minced

Fine sea salt

Freshly ground black pepper

3 cups low-sodium chicken or vegetable stock

1 carrot, peeled and chopped

1 bunch kale, stemmed and chopped

1 cup peeled and chopped sweet potato

1 cup filtered water

¼ teaspoon dried thyme

1 bay leaf

1. Coat the lamb cubes with tapioca flour. Put a tablespoon of ghee in a large soup pot over medium heat. Once the ghee is simmering, add the coated meat and brown it evenly.

2. Once the lamb is browned, add the onion, garlic, salt, and pepper. Sauté until the onion is fragrant. Add the stock and simmer for 30 to 35 minutes.

3. Add the carrot, kale, sweet potato, water, thyme, and bay leaf to the soup pot and simmer for 20 minutes, or until the vegetables are all tender.

4. Remove the soup from the heat and season with salt and pepper. Remove the bay leaf before serving.

Per Serving (1 bowl) Calories: 279; Total Fat: 10g; Saturated Fat: 3g; Sodium: 178mg; Carbohydrates: 22g; Fiber: 4g; Protein: 26g

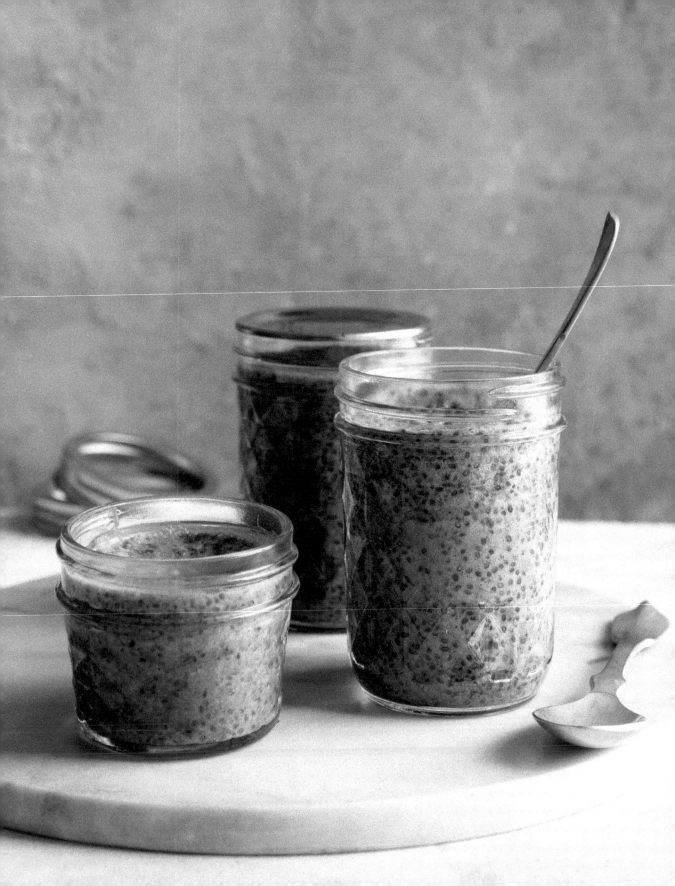

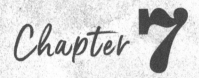

Snacks and Smoothies

Don't worry! Avoiding refined sugar and unhealthy fats does not mean banishing sweet and savory treats from your life. In this chapter, you'll find seven go-to recipes for satisfying midday and after-dinner cravings. Make big batches of your favorites ahead of time to keep yourself on the track to recovery.

No-Bake Banana Chocolate Chip Granola Bars

DAIRY-FREE, VEGETARIAN, VEGAN

The granola bars available at the grocery store may be convenient, but they're often loaded with added sugars and overpriced to boot! This simple recipe is a cost-effective way for you to make your own healthy granola bars at home. **YIELDS 12 BARS**

PREP TIME: 15 MINUTES (PLUS 1 HOUR TO CHILL)

2½ cups quick oats, uncooked

1 cup almond or cashew butter

½ cup pure maple syrup

¼ cup dried banana slices

¼ cup mini semisweet chocolate chips (my favorite dairy-free brand is Enjoy Life)

1. Line an 8-by-8-inch pan with parchment paper.

2. In a large bowl or food processor, combine the oats, nut butter, maple syrup, and dried banana. Mix thoroughly.

3. Add the chocolate chips and stir gently.

4. Transfer the batter into the lined pan and press firmly into place. Refrigerate for at least 1 hour, or until the batter has firmed up, before slicing into bars. Keep in the fridge for up to 2 weeks or in the freezer for up to 6 months.

Ingredient Tips: Choose unsulfured dried banana with no added sugar. If you need to eat gluten-free, use oats labeled specifically as gluten-free oats.

Per Serving (1 bar) Calories: 120; Total Fat: 5g; Saturated Fat: 1g; Sodium: 3mg; Carbohydrates: 17g; Fiber: 2g; Protein: 3g

Brain-Boosting Blueberry Smoothie

DAIRY-FREE, GLUTEN-FREE, VEGETARIAN, VEGAN

Smoothies make for a convenient snack and are a great way to sneak more vegetables into your diet! This smoothie contains blueberries, which have brain-protective properties, and kale, an excellent source of sulfur-based phytochemicals that upregulate your body's natural detoxification pathways. Make an extra effort to buy organic kale, if possible, since recent reports indicate that conventionally grown kale is unfortunately highly contaminated with pesticide residues. **SERVES 2**

PREP TIME: 10 MINUTES

⅔ cup frozen blueberries

1 frozen peeled banana

1 cup chopped kale leaves, fresh or frozen

2 tablespoons almond butter

½ cup full-fat coconut milk or almond milk

½ cup filtered water

Pure maple syrup or honey

In a blender, combine the blueberries, banana, kale, almond butter, coconut milk, water, and sweetener. Pulse until smooth and serve immediately.

Preparation Tip: Turn your smoothie into popsicles! Buy a silicone or stainless-steel popsicle mold and eat your brain-boosting smoothie as a popsicle. This is a great, healthy treat for enjoying all summer long.

Per Serving (1 smoothie or ½ recipe) Calories: 334; Total Fat: 24g; Saturated Fat: 14g; Sodium: 25mg; Carbohydrates: 31g; Fiber: 6g; Protein: 7g

Green Smoothie

DAIRY-FREE, GLUTEN-FREE, VEGETARIAN, VEGAN

We all know we should eat our greens but for some people this is easier said than done! If you're not a big fan of chewing your green vegetables, then this recipe is for you—it's loaded with kale and spinach and naturally sweetened with strawberries. Once you've tried this version, you'll find it easy to get in your greens! **SERVES 2**

PREP TIME: 2 MINUTES

1 cup unsweetened almond milk, plus more as needed

1 cup chopped kale leaves

1 cup fresh spinach leaves

6 strawberries, hulled

1 medium frozen peeled banana

1 tablespoon chia seeds

1 cup ice cubes

Place all the ingredients in a blender and blend until completely smooth. Add more nut milk to make a thinner smoothie.

Per Serving (1 smoothie or ½ recipe) Calories: 151; Total Fat: 4g; Saturated Fat: 1g; Sodium: 121mg; Carbohydrates: 27g; Fiber: 6g; Protein: 5g

Raspberry Chia Pudding

DAIRY-FREE, GLUTEN-FREE, VEGETARIAN, VEGAN

Chia seeds are considered a healthy fat with a dual purpose. These seeds help reduce inflammation and support cognitive function. Finally, a dessert that truly is good for you! SERVES 2

PREP TIME: 15 MINUTES

1 (13.5-ounce) can full-fat coconut milk

6 pitted Medjool dates

2 teaspoons vanilla extract

1 pint fresh or frozen raspberries

6 tablespoons chia seeds

1.   Put the coconut milk, dates, and vanilla in a blender and blend until completely smooth.

2.   Add the raspberries and blend again on low.

3.   Add the chia seeds, stirring instead of blending.

4.   Pour the chia pudding into glass jars, such as two glass Mason jars. Refrigerate for at least 6 hours, or until the pudding has thickened, before eating.

Ingredient Tip: This is a great recipe for adding some joint-supportive collagen protein. Add 1 to 2 scoops of collagen peptides when blending the coconut milk, dates, and vanilla to get a boost of protein. Note that adding these peptides makes the recipe no longer vegan or vegetarian.

Substitution Tips: Use "lite coconut milk" (lower in fat) or almond milk to reduce the calorie count. For a low-sugar alternative, you can substitute stevia or Lakanto monk fruit extract for the dates.

Per Serving (1 cup) Calories: 800; Total Fat: 61g; Saturated Fat: 42g; Sodium: 39mg; Carbohydrates: 117g; Fiber: 42g; Protein: 17g

Plantain Chips

DAIRY-FREE, GLUTEN-FREE, VEGETARIAN, VEGAN

Plantains are an excellent source of resistant starch, a type of dietary fiber that promotes the growth of beneficial bacteria in your gut. Plantain chips are a healthy, delicious alternative to less nutrient-dense options like potato and corn chips. **SERVES 3**

PREP TIME: 5 MINUTES
COOK TIME: 20 MINUTES

2 green plantains, peeled (avoid yellow or brown plantains, which may be too ripe to yield crispy chips)

2 tablespoons melted coconut oil or avocado oil

Fine sea salt

1. Preheat the oven to 375°F. Line a baking sheet with parchment paper.

2. Slice the plantains into ⅛-inch-thick slices using a very sharp knife or a mandoline cutter.

3. Lay the plantain slices on the baking sheet and drizzle with coconut oil and salt. Toss them gently to coat both sides with oil and salt.

4. Bake for 20 minutes, or until the plantains are crisp and a light golden brown on the edges. Flip once halfway through the baking process.

Serving Tip: Enjoy the plantain chips with guacamole, salsa, or hummus. They also taste great all by themselves!

Per Serving (1 ounce of chips or 10 to 25 chips, depending on size) Calories: 224; Total Fat: 10g; Saturated Fat: 8g; Sodium: 83mg; Carbohydrates: 38g; Fiber: 3g; Protein: 2g

Beet Hummus

DAIRY-FREE, GLUTEN-FREE, VEGETARIAN, VEGAN

This beet hummus is a magical pairing of two superfoods—chickpeas, which support the growth of beneficial gut bacteria, and beets, which are rich in micronutrients and a compound called betaine that supports your body's detoxification pathways. **SERVES 6**

PREP TIME: 15 MINUTES

1 roasted beet (see tip), cooled

1 (15-ounce) can chickpeas, rinsed
  and drained

Zest of 1 large lemon

Juice of 1 large lemon

2 garlic cloves minced

2 tablespoons tahini

¼ cup olive oil

Fine sea salt

Freshly ground black pepper

1. Place the beet in a food processor or blender and blend until almost completely smooth.

2. Add the chickpeas, lemon zest and juice, garlic, and tahini and blend until smooth.

3. Drizzle in the olive oil and mix by hand.

4. Transfer to a serving or storage dish and add salt and pepper to taste. The hummus can be stored in your refrigerator for up to 1 week.

Serving Tip: Enjoy this hummus with raw sliced veggies, whole-grain crackers, or Plantain Chips (page 122).

Ingredient Tip: You can find pre-roasted beets in the salad section of the grocery store. However, it is also really easy to cook them at home. To roast a beet, first peel it and chop it in halves or quarters. Roast it in a 425°F oven for 10 to 15 minutes, or until it is easily pierced with a knife.

Per Serving (¼ cup) Calories: 202; Total Fat: 13g; Saturated Fat: 2g; Sodium: 24mg; Carbohydrates: 18g; Fiber: 5g; Protein: 6g

Almond Butter Energy Balls

DAIRY-FREE, GLUTEN-FREE, VEGETARIAN, VEGAN

Energy balls are the perfect grab-and-go snack. You can make countless variations of this recipe using various nut butters and toppings such as coconut flakes, cacao powder, cacao nibs, and dried fruit. **YIELDS 18 ENERGY BALLS**

PREP TIME: 10 MINUTES (PLUS 35 TO 50 MINUTES TO CHILL)

1 cup unsweetened almond butter

⅓ cup pure maple syrup

½ cup almond flour or coconut flour

1. Line a small baking sheet or glass baking dish (one that will fit in your freezer or fridge) with parchment paper.

2. In a medium bowl or food processor, combine the almond butter, maple syrup, and flour and mix vigorously.

3. Place the energy ball "batter" in the fridge to firm up for 15 to 20 minutes.

4. Remove from the fridge and shape the batter into ping-pong-size balls.

5. Transfer the energy balls back to the fridge for 20 to 30 minutes, or until firm. Store in an airtight container in the fridge for up to 2 weeks.

Per Serving (1 energy ball) Calories: 125; Total Fat: 10g; Saturated Fat: 1g; Sodium: 37mg; Carbohydrates: 8g; Fiber: 2g; Protein: 4g

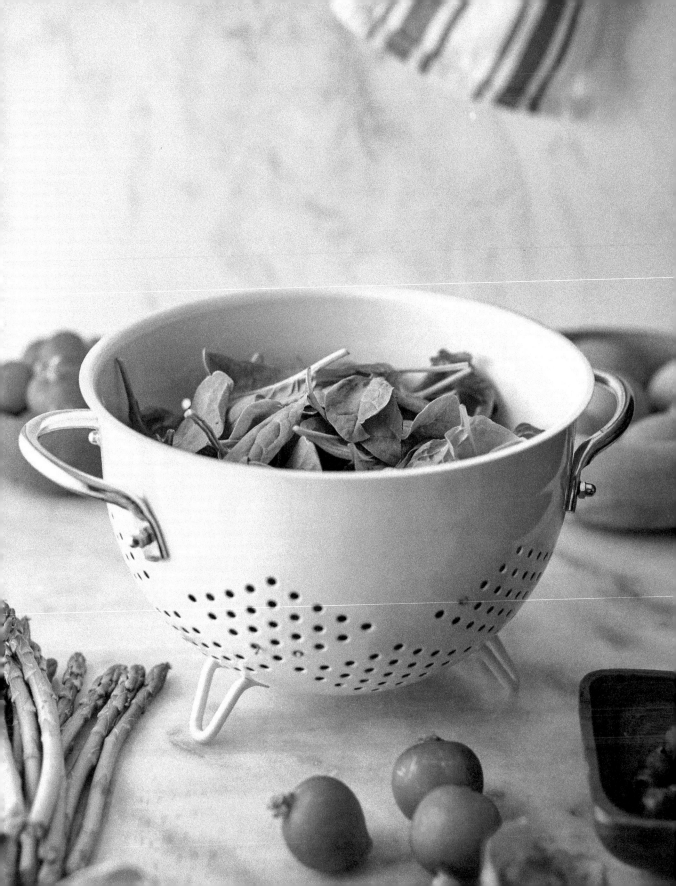

The Dirty Dozen and the Clean Fifteen™

A nonprofit environmental watchdog organization called the Environmental Working Group (EWG) looks at data supplied by the US Department of Agriculture (USDA) and the Food and Drug Administration (FDA) about pesticide residues. Each year it compiles a list of the best and worst pesticide loads found in commercial crops. You can use these lists to decide which fruits and vegetables to buy organic to minimize your exposure to pesticides and which produce is considered safe enough to buy conventionally. This does not mean it is pesticide-free, though, so wash these fruits and vegetables thoroughly. The list is updated annually, and you can find it online at EWG.org/FoodNews.

Dirty Dozen™

1. Strawberries
2. Spinach
3. Kale
4. Nectarines
5. Apples
6. Grapes
7. Peaches
8. Cherries
9. Pears
10. Tomatoes
11. Celery
12. Potatoes

Additionally, nearly three-quarters of hot pepper samples contained pesticide residues.

Clean Fifteen™

1. Avocados
2. Sweet corn*
3. Pineapples
4. Sweet peas (frozen)
5. Onions
6. Papayas*
7. Eggplants
8. Asparagus
9. Kiwis
10. Cabbages
11. Cauliflower
12. Cantaloupes
13. Broccoli
14. Mushrooms
15. Honeydew melons

*A small amount of sweet corn, papaya, and summer squash sold in the United States is produced from genetically modified seeds. Buy organic varieties of these crops if you want to avoid genetically modified produce.

Measurements and Conversions

	US STANDARD	US STANDARD (OUNCES)	METRIC (APPROXIMATE)
VOLUME EQUIVALENTS (LIQUID)	2 tablespoons	1 fl. oz.	30 mL
	¼ cup	2 fl. oz.	60 mL
	½ cup	4 fl. oz.	120 mL
	1 cup	8 fl. oz.	240 mL
	1½ cups	12 fl. oz.	355 mL
	2 cups or 1 pint	16 fl. oz.	475 mL
	4 cups or 1 quart	32 fl. oz.	1 L
	1 gallon	128 fl. oz.	4 L
VOLUME EQUIVALENTS (DRY)	⅛ teaspoon	———	0.5 mL
	¼ teaspoon	———	1 mL
	½ teaspoon	———	2 mL
	¾ teaspoon	———	4 mL
	1 teaspoon	———	5 mL
	1 tablespoon	———	15 mL
	¼ cup	———	59 mL
	⅓ cup	———	79 mL
	½ cup	———	118 mL
	⅔ cup	———	156 mL
	¾ cup	———	177 mL
	1 cup	———	235 mL
	2 cups or 1 pint	———	475 mL
	3 cups	———	700 mL
	4 cups or 1 quart	———	1 L
	½ gallon	———	2 L
	1 gallon	———	4 L
WEIGHT EQUIVALENTS	½ ounce	———	15 g
	1 ounce	———	30 g
	2 ounces	———	60 g
	4 ounces	———	115 g
	8 ounces	———	225 g
	12 ounces	———	340 g
	16 ounces or 1 pound	———	455 g

Resources

Books

Healing Lyme: Natural Healing of Lyme Borreliosis and the Coinfections Chlamydia and Spotted Fever Rickettsiosis, by Stephen Harrod Buhner

Stephen Harrod Buhner is a world-renowned herbalist with a deep, scientific interest in the use of botanical medicines for treating Lyme disease and Lyme disease coinfections. His book discusses which herbs are most useful for healing Lyme.

Why Can't I Get Better? Solving the Mystery of Lyme and Chronic Disease, by Dr. Richard I. Horowitz

This book is a must-read for anyone newly diagnosed with Lyme disease. It provides a revolutionary approach, developed by Dr. Horowitz, to treating complex, chronic illness.

Organizations and Websites

Bay Area Lyme Foundation

The Bay Area Lyme Foundation is an organization dedicated to developing methods for making Lyme disease easier to diagnose, and thus easier to treat.
https://www.bayarealyme.org/

Environmental Working Group

In addition to producing The Dirty Dozen and the Clean Fifteen™ lists that document levels of pesticides in produce, the Environmental Working Group also provides resources for selecting water filters and healthy personal care products. Together, the resources it provides can help you live an anti-inflammatory, healthy lifestyle.
https://www.ewg.org/

Global Lyme Alliance

Global Lyme Alliance is a nonprofit dedicated to conquering Lyme and other tick-borne diseases through increased awareness, research, and education.
https://globallymealliance.org/

International Lyme and Associated Diseases Society (ILADS)

ILADS is an organization that educates medical professionals about Lyme and associated diseases. It offers resources for helping patients find ILADS-certified, Lyme-literate doctors.
https://www.ilads.org/

ProHealth

ProHealth is an excellent resource for anti-inflammatory diet and lifestyle information specifically geared toward those with Lyme disease and other chronic illnesses.
https://www.prohealth.com/

Surviving Mold

Given the frequent co-occurrence of Lyme disease and mold illness, I recommend checking out the resources on this website to determine whether mold might be affecting your health.
https://www.survivingmold.com/

Thrive Market

Thrive Market is an online store that sells natural, healthy foods at prices much lower than Whole Foods and other health food stores. It is an excellent resource for buying many of the pantry items mentioned in this book.
https://thrivemarket.com

TickReport

TickReport allows you to send in a tick found on your body and carries out low-cost testing to determine whether it is carrying *B. burgdorferi* or other pathogens.
https://www.tickreport.com/

References

Chapter 1

Baker, Phillip J. "Perspectives on 'Chronic Lyme Disease.'" *The American Journal of Medicine* 121, no. 7 (2008): 562–564. doi:10.1016/j.amjmed.2008.02.013.

Bay Area Lyme Foundation. "Does Everyone Get the Telltale Bullseye Rash?" Accessed April 24, 2019. https://www.bayarealyme.org/blog/lyme-disease-bullseye-rash/.

Centers for Disease Control and Prevention. "How Many People Get Lyme Disease?" Accessed April 24, 2019. https://www.cdc.gov/lyme/stats/humancases.html.

Embers, Monica E., Nicole R. Hasenkampf, Mary B. Jacobs, Amanda C. Tardo, Lara A. Doyle-Meyers, Mario T. Philipp, and Emir Hodzic. "Variable Manifestations, Diverse Seroreactivity and Post-Treatment Persistence in Non-Human Primates Exposed to *Borrelia Burgdorferi* by Tick Feeding." *PLoS One* 12, no. 12 (2017): e0189071. doi:10.1371/journal.pone.0189071.

Johns Hopkins Medicine. "Study Shows Evidence of Severe and Lingering Symptoms in Some after Treatment for Lyme Disease." Accessed April 24, 2019. https://www.hopkinsmedicine.org/news/newsroom/news-releases/study-shows-evidence-of-severe-and-lingering-symptoms-in-some-after-treatment-for-lyme-disease.

Maxmen, Amy. "Antibodies Linked to Long-Term Lyme Symptoms." *Nature.* Accessed April 24, 2019. https://www.nature.com/news/2011/110805/full/news.2011.463.html.

Melia, Michael T., and Paul G. Auwaerter. "Time for a Different Approach to Lyme Disease and Long-Term Symptoms." *The New England Journal of Medicine* 374 (2016): 1277–1278. doi:10.1056/NEJMe1502350.

Moore, Andrew, Christina A. Nelson, Claudia Molins, Paul S. Mead, and Martin Schriefer. "Current Guidelines, Common Clinical Pitfalls, and Future Directions for Laboratory Diagnosis of Lyme Disease, United States." *Emerging Infectious Diseases* 22, no. 7 (2016). https://wwwnc.cdc.gov/eid/article/22/7/15-1694_article.

Nigrovic, Lise E., Desiree N. Neville, Fran Balamuth, Jonathan E. Bennett, Michael N. Levas, and Aris C. Garro. "A Minority of Children Diagnosed with Lyme Disease Recall a Preceding Tick Bite." *Ticks and Tick-borne Diseases* 10, no. 3 (2019): 694–696. doi:10.1016/j.ttbdis.2019.02.015.

Oosting, Marije, Mariska Kerstholt, Rob Ter Horst, Yang Li, Patrick Deelen, Sanne Smeekens, et al. "Functional and Genomic Architecture of *Borrelia burgdorferi*-Induced Cytokine Responses in Humans." *Cell Host & Microbe* 20, no. 6 (2016): 822–833. doi:10.1016/j.chom.2016.10.006.

Waddell, Lisa A., Judy Greig, Mariola Mascarenhas, Shannon Harding, Robbin Lindsay, and Nicholas Ogden. "The Accuracy of Diagnostic Tests for Lyme Disease in Humans: A Systematic Review and Meta-analysis of North American Research." *PLoS One* 11, no. 12 (2016): e0168613 doi:10.1371/journal.pone.0168613.

Wright, William F., David J. Riedel, Rohit Talwani, and Bruce L. Gilliam. "Diagnosis and Management of Lyme Disease." *American Family Physician* 85, no. 11 (2012): 1086–1093. https://www.ncbi.nlm.nih.gov/pubmed/22962880?dopt=Abstract.

Chapter 2

Aga, Miho, Kanso Iwaki, Yasuto Ueda, Shimpei Ushio, Naoya Masaki, Shigeharu Fukuda, et al. "Preventive Effect of *Coriandrum sativum* (Chinese parsley) on Localized Lead Deposition in ICR Mice." *Journal of Ethnopharmacology* 77, no. 2–3 (2001): 203–208. https://www.ncbi.nlm.nih.gov/pubmed/11535365/.

Berndtson, Keith. "Chronic Inflammatory Response Syndrome: Overview, Diagnosis, and Treatment." Accessed April 24, 2019. https://www.survivingmold.com/docs/Berndtson_essay_2_CIRS.pdf.

Black, David S., and George M. Slavich. "Mindfulness Meditation and the Immune System: A Systematic Review of Randomized Controlled Trials." *Annals of the New York Academy of Sciences* 1373, no. 1 (2016): 13–24. doi:10.1111/nyas.12998.

Bouzid, Mohamed Amine, Edith Filaire, Régis Matran, Sophie Robin, and Claudine Fabre. "Lifelong Voluntary Exercise Modulates Age-Related Changes in Oxidative Stress." *International Journal of Sports Medicine* 39, no. 1 (2018): 21–28. doi:10.1055/s-0043-119882.

Brewer, Joseph H., Jack D. Thrasher, David C. Straus, Roberta A. Madison, and Dennis Hooper. "Detection of Mycotoxins in Patients with Chronic Fatigue Syndrome." *Toxins (Basel)* 5, no. 4 (2013): 605–617. doi:10.3390/toxins5040605.

Buffen, Kathrin, Marije Oosting, Yang Li, Thirumala-Devi Kanneganti, Mihai G. Netea, and Leo A. B. Joosten. "Autophagy Suppresses Host Adaptive Immune Responses toward *Borrelia burgdorferi*." *Journal of Leukocyte Biology* 100, no. 3 (2016): 589598. doi:10.1189/jlb.4A0715-331R.

Campbell, John P., and James E. Turner. "Debunking the Myth of Exercise-Induced Immune Suppression: Redefining the Impact of Exercise on Immunological Health across the Lifespan." *Frontiers in Immunology* 9 (2018): 648. doi:10.3389/fimmu.2018.00648.

Catterson, James H., Mobina Khericha, Miranda C. Dyson, Alec J. Vincent, Rebecca Callard, Steven M. Haveron, et al. "Short-Term, Intermittent Fasting Induces Long-Lasting Gut Health and TOR-Independent Lifespan Extension." *Current Biology* 28, no. 11 (2018): 1714–1724. doi:10.1016/j.cub.2018.04.015.

Cheng, Chia-Wei, Gregor B. Adams, Laura Perin L, Min Wei, Xiayying Zhou, Ben S. Lam, et al. "Prolonged Fasting Reduces IGF-1/PKA to Promote Hematopoietic-Stem-Cell-Based Regeneration and Reverse Immunosuppression." *Cell Stem Cell* 14, no. 6 (2014): 810–823. doi:10.1016/j.stem.2014.04.014.

Daschner, Alvaro. "An Evolutionary-Based Framework for Analyzing Mold and Dampness-Associated Symptoms in DMHS." *Frontiers in Immunology* 7 (2017). doi:672. 10.3389/fimmu.2016.00672.

Ebnezar, John, Roghuram Nagarathna, Bali Yogitha, and Hongasandra Romarao Nagendra. "Effects of an Integrated Approach of Hatha Yoga Therapy on Functional Disability, Pain, and Flexibility in Osteoarthritis of the Knee Joint: A Randomized Controlled Study." *The Journal of Alternative and Complementary Medicine* 18, no. 5 (2012): 463–472. doi:10.1089/acm.2010.0320.

Ehrenstein O. S., C. Ling, X. Cui, M. Cockburn, A. S. Park, F. Yu, J. Wu, and B. Ritz. "Prenatal and Infant Exposure to Ambient Pesticides and Autism Spectrum Disorder in Children: Population-Based Case-Control Study." *BMJ* 364 (2019): l962. doi:10.1136/bmj.l962.

Environmental Working Group. "State of American Drinking Water." Accessed April 24, 2019. https://www.ewg.org/tapwater/state-of-american-drinking-water.php.

Fahey, Jed W., W. David Holtzclaw, Scott L. Wehage, Kristina L. Wade, Katherine K. Stephenson, and Paul Talalay. "Sulforaphane Bioavailability from Glucoraphanin-Rich Broccoli: Control by Active Endogenous Myrosinase." *PLoS One* [online] (2015). doi:10.1371/journal.pone.0140963.

Fahey, Jed W., Yuesheng Zhang, and Paul Talalay. "Broccoli Sprouts: An Exceptionally Rich Source of Inducers of Enzymes that Protect against Chemical Carcinogens." *Proceedings of the National Academy of Sciences of the United States of America* 94, no. 19 (1997): 10367–10372. https://www.ncbi.nlm.nih.gov/pmc/articles/PMC23369/.

Goyal, Madhav, Sonal Singh, Erica M.S. Sibinga, Neda F. Gould, Anastasia Rowland-Seymour, Ritu Sharma, et al. "Meditation Programs for Psychological Stress and Well-Being: A Systematic Review and Meta-Analysis." *JAMA Internal Medicine* 174, no. 3 (2014): 357–368. doi:10.1001/jamainternmed.2013.13018.

Greeson, Jeffrey, Haley Zarrin, Moria J. Smoski, Jeffrey G. Brantley, Thomas R. Lynch, Daniel M. Webber, et al. "Mindfulness Meditation Targets Transdiagnostic Symptoms Implicated in Stress-Related Disorders: Understanding Relationships between Changes in Mindfulness, Sleep Quality, and Physical Symptoms." *Evidence-Based Complementary and Alternative Medicine* 2018, Article ID 4505191 (2018): 10 pages. doi:10.1155/2018/4505191.

Harvard Health Publishing. "How to Boost Your Immune System." Accessed May 9, 2019. https://www.health.harvard.edu/staying-healthy/how-to-boost-your-immune-system.

Hussain, Joy, and Marc Cohen. "Clinical Effects of Regular Dry Sauna Bathing: A Systematic Review." *Evidence-Based Complementary and Alternative Medicine* 2018 (2018): 1857413. doi:10.1155/2018/1857413.

Ibarra-Coronado, Elizabeth G., Ana Ma. Pantaleón-Martínez, Javier Velazquéz-Moctezuma, Oscar Prospéro-García, Mónica Méndez-Díaz, Mayra Pérez-Tapia, Lenin Pavón, and Jorge Morales-Montor. "The Bidirectional Relationship between Sleep and Immunity against Infections." *Journal of Immunology Research* 2015, Article ID 678164: 14 pages. doi:10.1155/2015/678164.

Jang, Joon Hwan, Hye Yoon Park, Ul Soon Lee, Kyung-Jun Lee, and Do-Hyung Kang. "Effects of Mind-Body Training on Cytokines and Their Interactions with Catecholamines." *Psychiatry Investigation* 14, no. 4 (2017): 483–490. doi:10.4306/pi.2017.14.4.483.

Jiang, Tingting, Xuejin Gao, Chao Wu, Feng Tian, Qiucheng Lei, Jingcheng Bi, et al. "Apple-Derived Pectin Modulates Gut Microbiota, Improves Gut Barrier Function, and Attenuates Metabolic Endotoxemia in Rats with Diet-Induced Obesity." *Nutrients* 8, no. 3 (2016): 126. doi:10.3390/nu8030126.

Kerstholt, Mariska, Hedwig Vrijmoeth, Ekta Lachmandas, Marije Oosting, Mihaela Lupse, Mirela Flonta, et al. "Role of Glutathione Metabolism in Host Defense against *Borrelia burgdorferi* Infection." *Proceedings of the National Academy of Sciences of the United States of America* 115, no. 10 (2018): E2320–E2328. doi:10.1073/pnas.1720833115.

Khotimchenko, Maxim, Irina Serguschenko, and Yuri Khotimchenko. "Lead Absorption and Excretion in Rats Given Insoluble Salts of Pectin and Alginate." *International Journal of Toxicology* 25, no. 3 (2006): 195–203. doi:10.1080/10915810600683291.

Kikuchi, Masahiro, Yusuke Ushida, Hirokazu Shiozawa, Rumiko Umeda, Kota Tsuruya, Yudai Aoki, Hiroyuki Suganuma, and Yasuhiro Nishizaki. "Sulforaphane-Rich Broccoli Sprout Extract Improves Hepatic Abnormalities in Male Subjects." *World Journal of Gastroenterology* 21, no. 43 (2015): 12457–12467. doi:10.3748/wjg.v21.i43.12457.

Kong, Ling Jun, Romy Lauche, Petra Klose, Jiang Hui Bu, Xiao Cun Yang, Chao Qing Guo, Gustav Dobos, and Ying Wu Cheng. "Tai Chi for Chronic Pain Conditions: A Systematic Review and Meta-Analysis of Randomized Controlled Trials." *Scientific Reports* 6 (2016): 25325. doi:10.1038/srep25325.

Landrigan, Philip J., and Fiorella Belpoggi. "The Need for Independent Research on the Health Effects of Glyphosate-Based Herbicides." *Environmental Health* 17, (2018): 51. doi:10.1186/s12940-018-0392-z.

Lardone, Anna, Marianna Liparoti, Pierpaolo Sorrentino, Rosaria Rucco, Francesca Jacini, Arianna Polverino, et al. "Mindfulness Meditation Is Related to Long-Lasting Changes in Hippocampal Functional Topology during Resting State: A Magnetoencephalography Study." *Neural Plasticity* 2018 (2018): 5340717. doi:10.1155/2018/5340717.

Liew, Winnie-Pui-Pui, and Sabran Mohd-Redzwan. "Mycotoxin: Its Impact on Gut Health and Microbiota." *Frontiers in Cellular and Infection Microbiology* 8 (2018): 60. doi:10.3389/fcimb.2018.00060.

McCarthy, Matthew W., David W. Denning, and Thomas J. Walsh. "Future Research Priorities in Fungal Resistance." *The Journal of Infectious Diseases* 216, Suppl. 3 (2017): S484–S492. doi:10.1093/infdis/jix103.

Medic, Goran, Micheline Wille, and Michiel E. H. Hemels. "Short- and Long-Term Health Consequences of Sleep Disruption." *Nature and Science of Sleep* 9 (2017): 151–161. doi:10.2147/NSS.S134864.

Mullington, Janet M., Norah S. Simpson, Hans K. Meier-Ewert, and Monika Haack. "Sleep Loss and Inflammation." *Best Practice and Research: Clinical Endocrinology and Metabolism* 24, no. 5 (2010): 775–784. doi:10.1016/j.beem.2010.08.014.

National Research Council. "Implementing Health-Protective Features and Practices in Buildings: Workshop Proceedings: Federal Facilities Council Technical Report #148." Last modified 2005. doi:10.17226/11233.

Nishio, Ryusuke, Hanuna Tamano, Hiroki Morioka, Azusa Takeuchi, and Atsushi Takeda. "Intake of Heated Leaf Extract of *Coriandrum sativum* Contributes to Resistance to Oxidative Stress via Decreases in Heavy Metal Concentrations in the Kidney." *Plant Foods for Human Nutrition* [Epub ahead of print] (2019). doi:10.1007/s11130-019-00720-2.

Ratnaseelan, Aarane M., Irene Tsilioni, and Theoharis C. Theoharides. "Effects of Mycotoxins on Neuropsychiatric Symptoms and Immune Processes." *Clinical Therapeutics* 40, no. 6 (2018): 903–917. doi:10.1016/j.clinthera.2018.05.004.

Roehrs, Timothy, Maren Hyde, Brandi Blaisdell, Mark Greenwald, and Thomas Roth. "Sleep Loss and REM Sleep Loss Are Hyperalgesic." *Sleep* 29, no. 2 (2006): 145–151. https://www.ncbi.nlm.nih.gov/pubmed/16494081.

Rosanoff, Andrea, Connie M. Weaver, and Robert K. Rude. "Suboptimal Magnesium Status in the United States: Are the Health Consequences Underestimated?" *Nutrition Reviews* 70, no. 3 (2012): 153–164. doi:10.1111/j.1753-4887.2011.00465.x.

Shojaie, Marjan, Farzane Ghanbari, and Nasrin Shojaie. "Intermittent Fasting Could Ameliorate Cognitive Function against Distress by Regulation of Inflammatory Response Pathway." *Journal of Advanced Research* 8, no. 6 (2017): 697–701. doi:10.1016/j.jare.2017.09.002.

Sleiman, Sama F., Jeffrey Henry, Rami Al-Haddad, Lauretta El Hayek, Edwina Abou Haidar, Thomas Stringer, et al. "Exercise Promotes the Expression of Brain Derived Neurotrophic Factor (BDNF) through the Action of the Ketone Body β-hydroxybutyrate." *eLife* 5 (2016): E15092. doi:10.7554/eLife.15092.

Smith, Marie-Caroline, Stephanie Madec, Emmanuel Coton, and Nolwenn Hymery. "Natural Co-Occurrence of Mycotoxins in Foods and Feeds and Their *in vitro* Combined Toxicological Effects." *Toxins (Basel)* 8, no. 4 (2016): 94. doi:10.3390/toxins8040094.

Ussery, Emily N., Janet E. Fulton, Deborah A. Galuska, Peter T. Katzmarzyk, and Susan A. Carlson. "Joint Prevalence of Sitting Time and Leisure-Time Physical Activity among US Adults, 2015–2016." *Journal of the American Medical Association* 320, no. 19 (2018): 2036–2038. doi:10.1001/jama.2018.17797.

Vickers, Andrew J., Emily A. Vertosick, George Lewith, Mugh MacPherson, Nadine E. Foster, Karen J. Sherman, et al. "Acupuncture for Chronic Pain: Update of an Individual Patient Data Meta-Analysis." *The Journal of Pain* 19, no. 5 (2018): 455–474. doi:10.1016/j.jpain.2017.11.005.

Wang, Xiang, Peihuan Li, Chen Pan, Lisha Dai, Yan Wu, and Yunlong Deng. "The Effect of Mind-Body Therapies on Insomnia: A Systematic Review and Meta-Analysis." *Evidence-Based Complementary and Alternative Medicine* 2019, Article ID 9359807 (2019): 17 pages. doi:10.1155/2019/9359807.

Wang, Xuewen, Julian Greer, Ryan R. Porter, Kamaljeet Kaur, and Shawn D. Youngstedt. "Short-Term Moderate Sleep Restriction Decreases Insulin Sensitivity in Young Healthy Adults." *Sleep Health* 2, no. 1 (2016): 63–68. doi:1016/j.sleh.2015.11.004.

Ward, Mary H., Rena R. Jones, Jean D. Brender, Theo M. de Kok, Peter J. Weyer, Bernard T. Nolan, Cristina M. Villaneuva, and Simone G. van Breda. "Drinking Water Nitrate and Human Health: An Updated Review." *International Journal of Environmental Research and Public Health* 15, no. 7 (2018): 1557. doi:10.3390/ijerph15071557.

Xiang, Anfeng, Ke Cheng, Xueyong Shen, Ping Xu, and Sheng Liu. "The Immediate Analgesic Effect of Acupuncture for Pain: A Systematic Review and Meta-Analysis." *Evidence-Based Complementary and Alternative Medicine* 2017, Article ID 3837194. doi:10.1155/2017/3837194.

Yoshida, Kazutaka, Yusuke Ushida, Tomoko Ishijima, Hiroyuki Suganuma, Takahiro Inakuma, Nobuhiro Yajima, Keiko Abe, and Yuji Nakai. "Broccoli Sprout Extract Induces Detoxification-Related Gene Expression and Attenuates Acute Liver Injury." *World Journal of Gastroenterology* 21, no. 35 (2015): 10091–10103. doi:10.3748/wjg.v21.i35.10091.

Zeidan, Fadel, Joseph A. Grant, Chris A. Brown, John G. Mchaffie, and Robert C. Coghill. "Mindfulness Meditation-Related Pain Relief: Evidence for Unique Brain Mechanisms in the Regulation of Pain." *Neuroscience Letters* 520, no. 2 (2012): 165–173. doi:10.1016/j.neulet.2012.03.082.

Zinedine, Abdellah, Jose Miguel Soriano, Juan Carlos Molto, and Jordi Manes. "Review on the Toxicity, Occurrence, Metabolism, Detoxification, Regulations and Intake of Zearalenone: An Oestrogenic Mycotoxin." *Food and Chemical Toxicology* 45, no. 1 (2007): 1–18. https://www.ncbi.nlm.nih.gov/pubmed/17045381.

Chapter 3

Ak, Nese O., Dean Cliver, and Charles Kaspar. "Cutting Boards of Plastic and Wood Contaminated Experimentally with Bacteria." *Journal of Food Protection* 57, no. 1 (1994): 16–22. https://jfoodprotection.org/doi/abs/10.4315/0362-028X-57.1.16.

Aprotosoaie, Ana Clara, Anca Miron, Adriana Trifan, Vlad Simon Luca, and Irina-Iuliana Costache. "The Cardiovascular Effects of Cocoa Polyphenols—An Overview." *Diseases* 4, no. 4 (2016): 39. doi:10.3390/diseases4040039.

Blusztajn, Jan Krzysztof, Barbara E. Slack, and Tiffany J. Mellott. "Neuroprotective Actions of Dietary Choline." *Nutrients* 9, no. 8 (2017): 815. doi:10.3390/nu9080815.

Daley, Cynthia, Amber Abbott, Patrick Doyle, Glenn Nader, and Stephanie Larson. "A Review of Fatty Acid Profiles and Antioxidant Content in Grass-Fed and Grain-Fed Beef." *Nutrition Journal* 9 (2010): 10. doi:10.1186/1475-2891-9-10.

DiNicolantonio, James J., and James H. O'Keefe. "Importance of Maintaining a Low Omega-6/Omega-3 Ratio for Reducing Inflammation." *Open Heart* 5, no. 2 (2018): e000946. doi:10.1136/openhrt-2018-000946.

Feng, Jie, Wanliang Shi, Judith Miklossy, Genevieve M. Tauxe, Conor J. McMeniman, and Ying Zhang. "Identification of Essential Oils with Strong Activity against Stationary Phase *Borrelia burgdorferi*." *Antibiotics* 7, no. 4 (2018): 89. doi:10.3390/antibiotics7040089.

Gorzynik-Debicka, Monika, Paulina Przychodzen, Francesco Cappello, Alicja Kuban-Jankowska, Antonella Marino Gammazza, Narcyz Knap, et al. "Potential Health Benefits of Olive Oil and Plant Polyphenols." *International Journal of Molecular Sciences* 19, no. 3 (2018): 686. doi:10.3390/ijms19030686.

Hites, R.A., J. A. Foran, D. O. Carpenter, M. C. Hamilton, B. A. Knuth, and S. J. Schwager. "Global Assessment of Organic Contaminants in Farmed Salmon." *Science* 303, no. 5655 (2004): 226–229. https://www.ncbi.nlm.nih.gov/pubmed/14716013/.

Javid, Ashkan, Nataliya Zlotnikov, Helena Pětrošová, Tian Tian Tang, Yang Zhang, Anil K. Bansal, et al. "Hyperglycemia Impairs Neutrophil-Mediated Bacterial

Clearance in Mice Infected with the Lyme Disease Pathogen." *PLoS One* 11, no. 6 (2016): e0158019. doi:10.1371/journal.pone.0158019.

Kim, B., V. M. Hong, J. Yang, H. Hyun, J. J. Im, J. Hwang, S. Yoon, and J. E. Kim. "A Review of Fermented Foods with Beneficial Effects on Brain and Cognitive Function." *Preventive Nutrition and Food Science* 21, no. 4 (2016): 297–309. doi:10.3746/pnf.2016.21.4.297.

Lee, Sunhye, Katherine I. Keirsey, Rebecca Kirkland, Zachary I. Grunewald, Joan G. Fischer, and Claire B. de La Serre. "Blueberry Supplementation Influences the Gut Microbiota, Inflammation, and Insulin Resistance in High-Fat-Diet–Fed Rats." *The Journal of Nutrition* 148, no. 2 (2018): 209–219. doi:10.1093/jn/nxx027.

Mehedint, Mihai G., and Steven Zeisel. "Choline's Role in Maintaining Liver Function: New Evidence for Epigenetic Mechanisms." *Current Opinion in Clinical Nutrition and Metabolic Care* 16, no. 3 (2013): 339–345. doi:10.1097/MCO.0b013e3283600d46.

Nobuyuki Ito, Masao Hirose, Akihiro Hagiwara, and Satoru Takahashi. (1990). "Carcinogenicity and Modification of Carcinogenic Response by Antioxidants." Antimutagenesis and Anticarcinogenesis Mechanisms II. *Basic Life Sciences*, vol. 52, 183–194. Springer, Boston, MA.

Peedikayil, F.C., V. Remy, S. John, T. P. Chandru, P. Sreenivasan, and G. A. Bijapur. "Comparison of Antibacterial Efficacy of Coconut Oil and Chlorhexidine on *Streptococcus mutans*: An *in vivo* Study." *Journal of International Society of Preventive & Community Dentistry* 6, no. 5 (2016): 447–452. https://www.ncbi.nlm.nih.gov/pubmed/27891311.

Pop, Anca, Bela Kiss, and Felicia Loghin. "Endocrine Disrupting Effects of Butylated Hydroxyanisole (BHA - E320)." *Clujul Medical* 86, no.1 (2013): 16–20. https://www.ncbi.nlm.nih.gov/pmc/articles/PMC4462476/.

Qin, Bolin, Kiran Panickar, and Richard Anderson. "Cinnamon: Potential Role in the Prevention of Insulin Resistance, Metabolic Syndrome, and Type 2 Diabetes." *Journal of Diabetes Science and Technology* 4, no. 3 (2010): 685–693. doi:10.1177/193229681000400324.

Rayan, Paran, Deborah Stenzel, and Pauline Ann McDonnell. "The Effects of Saturated Fatty Acids on *Giardia duodenalis* Trophozoites in vitro." *Parasitology Research* 97 (2005): 191–200. https://link.springer.com/article/10.1007/s00436-005-1432-5.

Reger, Mark A., Samuel T. Henderson, Cathy Hale, Brenna Cholerton, Laura D. Baker, G. S. Watson, et al. "Effects of β-hydroxybutyrate on Cognition in Memory-Impaired Adults." *Neurobiology of Aging* 25, no. 3 (2004): 311–314. https://www.sciencedirect.com/science/article/pii/S0197458003000873?via%3Dihub.

Rezac, Shannon, Car Reen Kok, Melanie Heermann, and Robert Hutkins. "Fermented Foods as a Dietary Source of Live Organisms." *Frontiers in Microbiology* 9 (2018): 1785. doi:10.3389/fmicb.2018.01785.

Saebyeol, Jang, Jianghao Sun, Pei Chen, Sukla Lakshman, Aleksey Molokin, James M. Harnly, et al. "Flavanol-Enriched Cocoa Powder Alters the Intestinal Microbiota, Tissue and Fluid Metabolite Profiles, and Intestinal Gene Expression in Pigs." *The Journal of Nutrition* 146, no. 4 (2016): 673–680. doi:10.3945/jn.115.222968.

Seleem, Dalia, Emily Chen, Bruna Benso, Vanessa Pardi, and Ramiro M. Murata. "*In vitro* Evaluation of Antifungal Activity of Monolaurin against *Candida albicans* Biofilms." *PeerJ* 4 (2016): e2148. doi:10.7717/peerj.2148.

Socci, Valentina, Daniela Tempesta, Giovambattista Desideri, Luigi De Gennaro, and Michele Ferrara. "Enhancing Human Cognition with Cocoa Flavonoids." *Frontiers in Nutrition* 4, no. 19 (2017). doi:10.3389/fnut.2017.00019.

Subash, Selvaraju, Musthafa Mohamed Essa, Samir Al-Adawi, Mushtaq A. Memon, Thamilarasan Manivasagam, and Mohammed Akbar. "Neuroprotective Effects of Berry Fruits on Neurodegenerative Diseases." *Neural Regeneration Research* 9, no. 16 (2014): 1557–1566. doi:10.4103/1673-5374.139483.

Turley, Alexandra E., Joseph W. Zagorski, and Cheryl E. Rockwell. "The Nrf2 activator tBHQ Inhibits T Cell Activation of Primary Human CD4 T Cells." *Cytokine* 71, no. 2 (2015): 289–295. https://www.sciencedirect.com/science/article/abs/pii/S1043466614005894?via%3Dihub.

Wang, Qiao-Ping, Duncan Browman, Herbert Herzog, and G. Gregory Neely. "Non-Nutritive Sweeteners Possess a Bacteriostatic Effect and Alter Gut Microbiota in Mice." *PLoS One* 13, no. 7 (2018): e0199080. doi:10.1371/journal.pone.0199080.

Yang, Hsiao-Ting, Jenn-Wei Chen, Jagat Rathod, Yu-Zhen Jiang, Pei-Jane Tsai, Yuan-Pin Hung, et al. "Lauric Acid Is an Inhibitor of *Clostridium difficile* Growth *in Vitro* and Reduces Inflammation in a Mouse Infection Model." *Frontiers in Microbiology* 8 (2017): 2635. doi:10.3389/fmicb.2017.02635.

Index

Acknowledgments

When I was a young adult, Lyme disease dismantled my life; I never would have thought that I would come full circle and end up writing a book about the nutritional healing of this illness. However, if there's anything I've learned along my Lyme disease journey, it's that life is full of wonderful surprises!

I would like to express my gratitude to all the talented, caring health professionals who listened to me and supported me throughout the most trying times in my journey with Lyme disease. You listened to me when no one else would. Your compassion gave me the courage to keep seeking answers and never give up, even in the face of seemingly insurmountable challenges.

To my parents, siblings, relatives, and close friends who loved and supported me throughout my journey—I wouldn't be where I am today without you. Even when I felt I had lost myself, you remained by my side, and I will be forever grateful to you.

To all the people out there struggling with Lyme disease—I know that life with Lyme disease may seem dark, scary, and lonely at times, but know that you are not alone. Healing is entirely possible.

About the Author

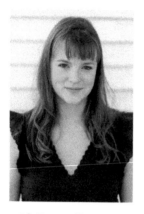 **Lindsay Christensen** has a bachelor's degree in biomedical science and a master's degree in human nutrition and is a proud health and science geek! Lindsay's passion for nutrition and health was shaped by her own battle with Lyme disease in her late teens and early twenties. When the conventional Lyme disease treatment approach failed, Lindsay took healing into her own hands. Thanks to the help of some wonderful doctors and many of the health strategies outlined in this book, Lindsay has recovered and now lives a full, healthy, and happy life. In her clinical nutrition practice, Ascent to Health, Lindsay helps clients with Lyme disease and other chronic illnesses restore their own health through evidence-based diet and lifestyle changes. In addition to working with clients, Lindsay performs research and writes for members of the healthcare industry, including Chris Kresser LLC and Quicksilver Scientific.

In her free time, Lindsay can be found outdoors rock climbing, hiking, running, and skiing. She also enjoys photographing her adventures and whipping up a healthy meal as soon as she gets home.

CPSIA information can be obtained
at www.ICGtesting.com
Printed in the USA
BVHW021340010819
554793BV00002B/2/P

9 781641 525565